Traditional Medicine Making of the 'Emu' –
Continuity and Change

Kingsley Ifeanyi Owete

Traditional Medicine Making of the 'Emu' – Continuity and Change

PL ACADEMIC RESEARCH

Bibliographic Information published by the Deutsche Nationalbibliothek
The Deutsche Nationalbibliothek lists this publication in the Deutsche Nationalbibliografie; detailed bibliographic data is available in the internet at http://dnb.d-nb.de.

Library of Congress Cataloging-in-Publication Data
Owete, Kingsley I. (Kingsley Ifeanyi), 1964- author.
Traditional medicine making of the 'Emu' : continuity and change / Kingsley Ifeanyi Owete.
pages cm
Includes bibliographical references.
ISBN 978-3-631-65978-6
1. Traditional medicine—Nigeria—Emu-Uno. 2. Ethnopharmacology—Nigeria—Emu-Uno. 3. Rites and ceremonies—Nigeria—Emu-Uno. 4. Emu-Uno (Nigeria)—Religion. I. Title.
GN477097 2015
615.8'809669--dc23
2015007143

ISBN 978-3-631-65978-6 (Print)
E-ISBN 978-3-653-05449-1 (E-Book)
DOI 10.3726/978-3-653-05449-1

PL Academic Research is an Imprint of Peter Lang GmbH.

Peter Lang – Frankfurt am Main · Bern · Bruxelles · New York · Oxford · Warszawa · Wien

This publication has been peer reviewed.

www.peterlang.com

Foreword

Despite the growth in science and technology, African traditional religion and practices continue to attract followership among Africans across all strata. Against this background, K. I. Owete's *Continuity and Change – Traditional Medicine Making in an Indigenous African Society* is an innovative research on the persistence and preference for traditional medical healing and protection on the part of many Africans. This book is a booster to the cognitive approach to the study of religion, dealing with the psychological and spiritual dimensions of traditional mode of healing and protection.

While there are many scholarly works on traditional medicine, their findings are mostly tainted with Christian biases. Contrarily, Owete makes an in-depth study of an ethnic group to explore traditional mode of protection, taxonomy, causality and therapy. He highlights the significance of ritual symbolism in the belief and practice of medicine making in the indigenous African society of Emu.

This book would be of immense benefit to religious scholars, cognitive theorists, policy makers on traditional medicine making, and general audience interested in African cultures.

Prof. W. O Wotogbe-Weneka
Department of Religious and Cultural Studies
University of Port Harcourt, Nigeria
March, 2014.

Acknowledgements

The research for this book brought me in contact with a number of people whose contributions deserve my sincere acknowledgment. I am indebted to my wife, Chinwe Owete for her companionship, moral and spiritual assistance in the course of researching and writing this book.

My colleagues at the University of Port Harcourt, Choba, assisted me in various ways. I want to recognize the critical comments and astute remarks of Professors C. I. Ejizu, E. S. Akanma, V. G. Nyayoko, W. O. Wotagbe-Weneka and A. R. O. Kilani. I owe Prof. Femi Shaka a debt of gratitude for taking time to read through the drafts. I shall not fail to thank Prof. Robin Horton, whose guidance and borrowed books, helped in sharpening the thoughts expressed in this book.

A special commendation also goes to Dr. Maxwell Iwegbue and Dr. Nicholas Alumona, they helped with the translations of Ukwuani words and phrases contained in the book. I appreciate my younger brother, Azubike Owete for making numerous trips to Emu Unor to make arrangements for interview in the course of researching for this book. Finally, I am thankful to my little brother, Dr. Jones U. Odili who fondly read through the draft manuscript and offered publication advice. Thanks to all informants listed in the appendix.

Most of all, I want to give thanks to the Lord for all He has done for me. This work would not have been done if not for God's hands that have always been upon me.

I take full responsibility for all errors and omissions in this work.

K. I. Owete
March, 2014

Table of Contents

Chapter One

1.1 Overview

In 1986, General Olusegun Obasanjo advocated the use of traditional medicine to dismantle the oppressive apartheid regime in South Africa. In March 1977, at Benin City, the Nigerian Army held a seminar to which indigenous medicine men were invited. The aim of the meeting was to explore the possibility of tapping the potentials inherent in African traditional medicines, for military and defence purposes (Fabarebo, 1990: 3). Around 1987, universities in Sokoto and Bendel (now split into Edo and Delta states) States were employing "juju" men to solve what they considered as intractable problems. After the Vice Chancellor of one of the institutions was bitten by a mysterious snake, the school sought the assistance of medicine men to rid the school of snakes. In another development at Bendel State University (now Ambrose Alli University Ekpoma), the thieves that carted away the university property were detected and apprehended by the use of traditional medicine (Fabarebo, 1990: 8). In 1990, the news was widespread in respect of two undergraduate students of the University of Jos who became victims to ritual medicine. Unknown to one of them, a female student, her father had laced her with "*magun alemaro*". This medicine is to make turgid the penis of whoever tries to have sex with her. However, the male lover decided to use his tongue instead (cunnilingus). The tongue and the head of the boy increased tremendously and then exploded. The above instances speak to the reality of the belief in ritual medicine. The question is why do we (Nigerians) still engage in traditional medicine and why does the belief still continue in our society, despite the perceived collapse of traditional beliefs and practices? These questions owe in part to the pursuit and the re-discovery of the African traditional medicine in the 21st century.

In an attempt to introduce research into traditional medicine, the University of Ibadan (African Studies Institute) established degree programs in African Traditional Medicine. This and other institutional undertakings are serious efforts to uncover values in medicinal plants that are becoming increasingly viable as more and more diseases are showing resistance to orthodox antibiotics, the side effects of which are of a great medical concern. This concern accounts for the recent move away from the use of synthetic medicine to galenicals and the use of herbs which form about 90% of the traditional medicine (Ubrurhe, 2003: 1). Against this backdrop, the quest of this work was to investigate the religious beliefs and rituals of Emu people, with the view of documenting their medicinal practices within the context of change.

Where new influences infringe on any society, a scholar of culture is at once confronted with the problem of how much is modified and how much is retained (Bascom & Herskovitz, 1959: 06). Consequent upon the aggressive wind of change that heralded capitalistic penetration in Africa, the boundaries of the old ethnic kingdoms were shattered. Indigenous beliefs, ideas, practices and norms that were held sacrosanct and sacred were almost obliterated. The impact of the drastic shift from traditional collectivism to individualism and from spiritualism to materialism is profound. This shift is the main focus of this book.

Existing literatures in African religions (in general) including traditional medicine tend to be dominated by data obtained from small – scale societies. The cultural anthropologists who initially researched this field studied religion within structuralism and functionalism. These approaches may be useful for the study of distinctive religio-cultural elements such as medicine, sorcery, witchcraft, and rites of passage. However, among the Emu people, such studies were carried out in a sweeping fashion lacking analysis on continuity and change. Additionally, historical and phenomenological studies have been absent. In view of the above limitation, the goals of this book are:

1. To provide a systematic and descriptive documentation of indigenous beliefs and practices of the Emu people.
2. To examine the relationship between Emu contemporary economic and socio-political situations in the context of continuity and changes to the people's religious beliefs and ritual practices concerning medicine.
3. To use the facts from Emu as basis for examining changes and consequences of religious changes in Africa.

1.2 Approach

Given the systemic inquiry that the study of this book adopts, there is a heavy dependence on the Husserlina principles of understanding-epoch, eidetic vision, empathy and quest from meaning. This theoretical perspective makes it possible to avoid the cold objectivity that defines western scholarly approach. Ayward Shorter in his book, *African Christian Theology* (1975: 39), listed eight approaches which have been adopted by different authors in the study of African religions. Out of these eight, he suggested that the multidimensional approach-historical, limited comparative, categorical and thematic approaches will be better suited to the study of African religions.

Harold Turner argued against Short's multidimensional approaches. For Turner, religion is a "human activity and experience that is liable to be inter-woven with all aspects of human life, and its study therefore requires, sooner or later, all human science" (Turner, 1981: 1–2). In the study of religion, the methods employed should, according to him, be able "to study, not only religion in its total milieu and that milieu itself, but also what it is that is interwoven with all other dimensions of existence". Shorter's approach, according to Ikenga-Metuh, is an anthropological study of African Religions, which may be useful for the study of the milieu of religion but inadequate for the study of the distinctive elements of religions. Ikenga-Metuh further noted that "in the four approaches that make up Shorter's Multidimensional method, no mention was made of the specialist religious disciplines" (Metuh, 1987: 87). This book marks the first attempt to study the traditional religion of the Emu people with specific focus on its' specialists use of herbs or practice of medicine. The major approach is documentation of practices as well as descriptive description of the practices underscoring the importance of the medicines that are used within the contexts in which they are used.

1.3 Terminologies

Of importance to this work are certain concepts and terms such as tradition, medicine, and traditional medicine. Since these terms will feature prominently in this work, and because there are certain negative stereotypes associated with them it is important to make clear the manner in which they are used. Tradition refers to doctrine, belief, opinion, custom, and story that is passed from generation to generation, especially orally. By medicine is meant any object, spell or rite that is supposed to have natural or supernatural powers as a remedy or curative. There are ritual medicines that are used for the cure of diseases. Most times, these ritual medicines involve the use of incantations alongside the medicinal substance. It is common place to say that the efficacy of the medicine is dependent on both the active ingredients of the ritual medicine and the incantations. This fact has been acknowledged in the definition of medicine by Parrinder (1969: 156), who stated that medicine in the African context covers both natural healing agencies such as leaves and roots, and the invocations of ritual or spiritual influence that are thought to be associated with them. It includes anything that can be used to heal, kill, to secure power, health, fertility, personality or moral reforms (Metuh, 1985). *Igwo Ogwu* (medicine making) includes the use of herbal, psychotherapeutical and spiritual techniques. Medicine includes herbal mixtures, ritual objects, incantations and rites capable of changing the human condition for better or worse (Metuh, 1985: 162).

Traditional medicine is the method of healing or curing diseases as well as preventing diseases, which have been handed down from generation to generation. It is the oral transmission of the knowledge and practices, based on customary methods of natural healing or treatment of disease (Mume, n.d.: 27). It is also the total combination of knowledge and practice, whether explicable or not, used in diagnosing, preventing or eliminating a physical, mental or social disease which may rely exclusively on past experience and observation handed down from generation to generation, verbally or in writing (Sofowora, 1984: 21).

An important distinction has to be made between "medicine" and "ritual medicine". Ritual medicines involve the use of incantations for the treatment, prevention or cure of diseases; it is difficult to say whether the efficacy of ritual medicine is in the active ingredients or in the incantations. Contrarily, medicine is a cover term for natural healing agencies such as leaves, roots and the invocation of ritual or spiritual influences that are thought to be associated with them (Parrinder, 1965: 69). It is also anything that can be used to heal, kill, and secure power, health, fertility, personality or moral reforms. Medicine thus includes drugs for curing and preventing disease as well as objects with ritual effects (Metuh, 1987: 7). Finally, there is the making of medicine (*Igwo ogwu*) as well as psycho-therapeutical and spiritual techniques. The making of medicine is not limited to herbal mixtures; it includes ritual objects, incantations, and rites capable of changing the human conditions for the better or worse (Metuh, 1986: 162).

Chapter Two: Theories of Change

There is a significant amount of scholarly interest in religious beliefs and ritual practices in general. Within and outside of the African continent there are theoretical views and models of religious change in response to the increase in knowledge and the refinement of the means to studying cultures. This chapter examines change in African traditional religion. This will be followed by an introduction of the Ukwuani traditional religion.

2.1 Religious Belief and Ritual Practices

Two anthropological schools have generated a great deal of material published on religious beliefs and ritual in Africa. These are the British and the French schools. The British school was primarily interested in the sociological aspect of religious belief and ritual practices. Specifically, they focused on the causal link between disturbed social relations and disease or misfortune. Religious beliefs and ritual practices were investigated more as functional components in the social machinery than in their own right as a phenomenon. The French school on the other hand focused on the symbolic-philosophical order and regarded it as the determinant of both social structure and African life, i.e., law, ethics, psychology and ritual (Ikenga-Metuh, 1987: 76).

In the 1970s, scholars of African traditional religions began to develop more critical historical approaches to the study of African indigenous religion (due to the influence of Evans Pritchards who wrote on Nuer religion). Ranger and Kimambo in their editor's introduction to 'the historical study of African Religion: with special Reference to East and central Africa (1972: 7), suggested that the main problem in the study of African Traditional Religion is that most scholars have seen the religion as having an eternal and unchanging outlook and have made an erroneous assumption that religious change did not occur. Ranger and Kimambo advocate a historical study of African Traditional Religion and argue that, it should proceed along the same lines as the historical study of, for instance, precolonial systems. The use of archive, oral evidence, linguistics and archaeological evidence should be adopted.

Robin Horton (1971) in his article "African Conversion" shows how, in the mainly unelaborated idea of the Supreme Being and other areas, the traditional religions had great adaptive potential. He further shows how, in the face of the challenges of social change commerce, education, science, technology, "people do not abandon their traditional cosmology rather they re-mold and develop it until it attains once more its pristine level of explanatory coverage" (1971: 45).

Okechuku Okeke, in his "Religious Change in Ikenagzizi" (1982: 16), appraised the nature of religious change in a Igboland, says that long before the coming Christianity, some people had abandoned old deities and cults which they saw no longer relevant and accepted new spirits, gods and institutions that appeared more relevant. He cited an instance where *Amadioha*, a god of thunder and lightning, from Igboland, was adopted in Ikwerreland before the advent of Christianity. Cyril Okorocha (1987) re-echoed Okeke's assertion that religious change among the Igbo occurred mainly to satisfy people's needs at particular times. According to him, those gods seen as not fulfilling peoples' needs were either abandoned or given new functions to meet these needs. These works are in agreement on the change to religion and the selective nature of the changes. These works also emphasized the idea of innovation, as well as replacement of old gods with new ones to meet new needs, or rebranding of them and giving to them new functions.

2.2 Social Change and religion

The origin, causes, patterns, influences and consequences of change within societies have justifiably been the preoccupations of scholars in the fields of contemporary African sociology and social anthropology. Okaba (1996) observed that the search for theories of social change in contemporary Africa must be premised first, on a critical assessment of existing explanations of change as they have been applied to the continent and considered unique to society. However, any significant discourse on the issue of religion and cultural changes will have to be focused on the identification of or/and explanation of causality and the processes of change, in addition to the relationship between religious and other cultural institutions. There are two important types of change, namely organizational change and behavioral change that occurs when there is a transformation among the parts of an institution. Understanding the distinction between them enables one to assess the level of continuity and discontinuity in African social life.

According to Ikenga-Metuh (1986: 46) the causes of religio-cultural change are many and varied. He categorized these into religious conviction and activities, such as the reformatory, revivalist, and syncretistic influence of Christianity and Islam on indigenous cultures in Nigeria. Non-religious factor such as political factors, for instance, political conquest and colonialism that include changes in the economic system (e.g. mode of production) and socio-structural changes such as urbanization and sophistication in science and technology. However, the boundaries and spheres of influence of these agents are not water-tight, rather they over-lap. The interactionists would on the above premise see the inter-mingling of various religious doctrines and faith within the same social-cultural population as a catalyst of change. With respect to patterns of religious changes, mention has to be made of the dualistic typology. It derives its basic assumption from the modernization theory of development which is also referred to as the theory of process. According to Scanzoni and Scanzoni (1978: 6), the dualistic typology presumes that all developments lead to transformation progress, diversification, complexity and social modernization.

2.3 Theories of Religious Change

Baike (1856) described the religion of Ukwani people, whom he had referred to as the Igbo of Aboh, as entirely "pagan", mixed up with numerous rites and ceremonies, neither in general so frightful nor so bloody as those practiced in Bini, in Dahomey, and other western countries, but still all of a pre-eminently superstitious character. This assertion is line with the early western anthropologist goal of studying traditional religions not for their own sake, as a subject, but to give a demonstration of what primitive religion looked like. The author's concern was to show Ukwuani people as primitive people with primitive religion and this is evidenced by his lexical choices. For instance, he used the phrase "entirely pagan" to describing the religion of the Ukwuani people. Of course, the word "pagan" like "fetishism", "animism", "juju", "savage", are derogatory and unsuitable words in describing Ukwuani Traditional Religion or the religion of any African group.

Unegbu (1954: 66) while describing the religion of Ukwuani people, claimed that the strange thing was that the place was full of "idols", and an altar of worship was dedicated to any god that claimed to exercise some influenced over man, but there was none to the "Unknown God of the Greek" or the "Great god" of the Igbos. Rev. Unegbu's description of Ukwuani Religions seems to be that of a scholar in two worlds. That is, the world of European missionaries and a world of African theologians. Firstly, the author's concern was not to describe Ukwuani religion phenomenological, but to replace it with Christianity. This, he tried to do in two ways, discontinuity and continuity. Firstly, the author uses strong language like "idols" to present the religion in a negative way such that the adherents would desert it. Unegbu further tries to show that Christianity has come to compliment African traditional religion as Christ says that he has "come to build and not to destroy". Arguing against this approach, Okot p'Bitek (1971) said that the missionaries painted a false image of African traditional religion. He concluded that either discontinuity or continuity the missionaries are using African Traditional Religion as a mercenary in a foreign battle. Furthermore Unegbu like the apologist of his time appealed to Greek philosophy in his description of Ukwuani religion by invoking categories and concepts that are all abstract to the local people, namely the "Unknown God" and the "Great God".

No society should be seen as static. The organic parts of any society change not necessarily in a unilinear fashion. Since all segments are interconnected, it is only through a process of the interplay between these parts that change occurs. These changes are either catalyzed by internal strain or by external agents. However, any discussion on the subject of change is not complete or conclusive without an assessment of the degree of continuity itself. The pro-modernization model see religious change in Africa as the outcome of the displacement of subdued primitive, passive, indigenous, social and religious structures by dominant, modern, dynamic, colonial and missionary social and religious structures. The indigenous models on the other hand recognize the continuity of traditional belief amidst the aggressive force of change. African religious and cultural institutions are die-hards.

African cosmology is adaptive and thus capable of changing according to evolving circumstance and times. Therefore, for any model to adequately explain the uniqueness of the nature of change found in Africa, it must duly recognize the elements of change and continuity. It should also take a look at the prevalent mode of production to properly articulate causal agents, relationship, processes and consequences of change in African societies. Intrinsic in this model, is the organic structure of a society. Little wonder the structural-functionist theory of change is seen as the theoretical foundation for modernization perspectives. Religion has largely been seen as a social tool for evolution. Durkheim (1935: 108) who subscribes to this school of thought posited that "as society evolves, her clan units change because religion is a unified system of beliefs and practice, by which individuals represent to themselves the society to which they belong and their relation to it". Durkheim further touches on the importance of religion as a cosmology by offering an explanation of the natural, social and supernatural world. And he came down on the social function of religious ritual in creating a feeling of solidarity among participants as well as an awareness of the reality greater than themselves which he felt was functional for social discipline.

In consonance with the foregoing tradition, Parsons (1951) approaches the problem of change in the context of social structures, social order, and social system. For him, social systems are action systems operating within cultural, personality and physical environments. These systems tend to be in equilibrium. The sub-units of society emerge to satisfy four basic problems: adaptation goal, attainment, integration and pattern maintenance. Changes never affect these basic functions because they possess capability for continual differentiation (Parsons, 1951: 64–68). Parsons (1951: 67). He further notes that change is evolutionary and appreciable so long as it enhances the adaptive capacity of the system. It is unacceptable if it disrupts the equilibrium already in the place. Max Weber (1963; 1964) examines the relationship between ideology and social action and how a change in the former can lead to change in the latter. In his opinion, social group ideas are developed on the basic tenets of their religion and its implication for their economic activities. Perhaps, his most important work in this area is the *Protestant Ethics and the Spirit of Capitalism* (1958). In it, he argues that although shared religious beliefs might integrate social groups, they may in turn have repercussions which, on the long run, can produce change in the economic, political and social contexts.

Dennis (1980) using Nigeria as a case study, examines how religious change has led to the complete transformation of its economic and political structure. She tries to show that a person's religious belief and conviction could have an effect on his/her economic activities. Influenced by Weber, Dennis noted that, "…for traders Islam has provided a set of belief about the conduct of trade, a social network and source of credit which enable them to expand the area which they trade (African Agege). Their economic enterprise was clearly related to their desire for religious independence…" (Dennis, 1980: 154–550). She concludes that, one of the most striking examples in which religious belief may affect economic behavior is found in the community of Aiyetoro founded on the biblical idea of systematic work and communal living (Dennis, 1980: 160).

According to Ikenga-Metuh (1985: 16–20) the dualistic typology and its functionalist perspective demonstrates that religion, though emerged as a dependent variable, that is an invention of society, has evolved to assume the status of an independent variable, possessing the potential of propelling change. Thus, religio-cultural structures, institutions, rites, behavior and values are not static but dynamic with the society – i.e., changing the ingredient of the culture and also being changed in the process. Humphrey Fisher (1973: 3) stressed that religious changes within a society, like conversion in a group or among individuals, is a process with which various stages could be identified. The first stage according to him is the state of adhesion. This is a period where novices to the new religion still maintain aspects of their old religion and aspects of their new religion. This stage leads to the second, the "stage of mixing" and finally to the stage of full conviction. He contends that with the obvious syncretization of belief systems in most indigenous society, most of the supposed converts are still at the level of adhesion in spite of the mass drift from the traditional religion to Islam or Christianity.

Finally, there is the Marxian conflict model to religious-cultural change. This model views religious institutions and other cultural correlates as the product of material consciousness. For Marx, a person's consciousness is determined by his\her social existence and the real dynamics of change is a person's action in shaping his\her existential reality. The mode of production in material life determines the general character of social, political and ideological process of life (Ake, 1980: 18). Marx disagrees with the functionalist consensus model of change, which sees religion as a catalyst of change. He argues rather, that the degree or pattern of religious change in society is the function of the model of production. Life is not determined by our consciousness rather it is our consciousness that is determined by life. Economic factors exert primary influence and largely shape other aspects of man and society. It is often argued that Marx's view of history and change is premised on the ideology of the dialectics. Social change is not a smooth and orderly progression which gradually unfolds in harmonious evolution. Instead, it proceeds from contradictions built into society which are sources of tension and ultimately the root of conflict and radical change. The Marxian postulation also demonstrates how change could occur in response to internal strain or to other dysfunctional elements as well as in confrontation with intruding external change agents (Haralambos, 1980: 534–540).

Different from the preceding are some theories of religious change with focus and analysis that are predicated on African situations. Foremost is the socio-structuralist explanation which generally sees non-religious factors as being responsible for change in African religious institutions. A protagonist of this model, Triminghan (1955), ascribes the large scale religious change during the colonial and post-colonial epochs to the resultant collapse of the traditional society. With this collapse, he claimed, came the consequent collapse of the traditional religious system that is closely tied to it. For him, since the traditional world views that were intended for a microcosmic village and clan life could not sustain experiences to which it is now exposed; Africans had no choice but to adopt one of the new religious systems, with a universal world view-Christianity or Islam.

The intellectualist model propounded by Horton (1971: 102) is an extension of the foregoing. Central to the intellectualist model is that conversion from traditional religious beliefs and practices to those of the world evangelical religions occurs in response to the changes in social organization. He observed that if thousands of people find themselves outside the microcosm, and if even those left inside see the boundaries weakening, if not actually dissolving, they can only interpret these changes by assuming that the lesser spirits are in retreat. A careful examination of Horton's thesis reveals that, he did not consider change to be mono-causal. In his opinion, change is not entirely caused by external agents as postulated by the dualistic topologists. He relates change in the indigenous cosmology and the social structure to change in the religious belief system. Horton goes on note that those who got converted into new religions with hope of greater socio-political benefits were disappointed. The resultant disillusionments produce religious syncretism.

2.4 Religious Changes and African Traditional Religion

It has been observed that for more than half a century, the missionary onslaught had not completely led to the routing and retreating of the traditional gods, Ejizu (1986: 134). Rather, "the introduction of Christianity has given religious choice and characteristically; many Igbo have accepted Christianity without rejecting their traditional religious beliefs" Ottenberg (1959: 55). Similar observation was made by Bascom and Herskovits (1959: 45) that:

> Despite the intensity of Christian missionary efforts...which have marked the history of various parts of Africa, African religions continue to manifest vitality everywhere. This is to be seen on the worship of African deities, the homage to the ancestors and the recourse to divination, medicine and other rituals.

The traditional concept of time in Africa *Zamani* (referring to the glorious past) and *Sasa* (referring to the present and vague future), is totally bound up with the life of the people and its comprehension may show the thinking, attitude and actions of African people Mbiti (1969: 23). Mbiti goes on to state that the traditional organization, where the African idea of time is two-dimensional, makes human life largely stable and almost static. He says that radical change is not known, not acceptable or so slow that is not noticed. According to him, changes that occurred were due to the emergence of European missionaries from the mid-nineteenth century with their civilization including Christianity. Mbiti's concept of time is not applicable to all African societies neither is his assertion that Christianity and western civilization were instrumental to changes in the traditional religions. Africans have been changing those areas of their religion which seem to need adjustments. Christianity and civilization only sped up the process.

Idowu (1973) whilst looking at the problems besetting the study of African Traditional religions suggested that the influence of other cultures and religions is significant in Africa. In contact between Africans and other cultures, African people either forget their traditional religions or combine their practices with the new religions Idowu (1973: 38). Thus, Idowu painted a picture of the African Traditional religion as a dying or dead religion while seeing other religions as dynamic. Finally, African Traditional Religions have the capacity of elaboration of the idea of the Supreme Being even before the emergence of Christianity and Islam due to the expansion of their microcosmic view to a wider macrocosmic view as a result of commerce, Fisher (1975).

2.5 Modern Changes in African Traditional Religions

There are numerous scholarly documentation of different of cultural and religious changes for many societies. One way in which people respond to new challenges in pre-modern times was not by searching for new gods, but calling upon existing gods to take up new tasks (Horton, 1962: 19). The making new demands of old gods is not arbitrary, rather it occurs in light of the peoples' knowledge of the god's existing capabilities. An example cited by Horton is *Ojoye Adum* a deity among the people of Orusangama in the eastern part of Niger Delta. At the time of Horton's stay in Orusangama, the people engaged in fishing, hunting, subsistence agriculture and made produce from raffia palm. They exported surpluses from these activities upstream where they exchanged their goods for dry land food stuffs. The most important water spirit was *Duminea*. The spirit owned very large areas that included not only the territorial waters of Orusangama but also those of the powerful neighboring village of Soku. Orusangama people acted as junior partners to Soku in rites addressed to the spirit. However, some years before Horton arrived in Orusangama, a new water spirit announced itself by possessing a man. This spirit said that its' name was *Ojiye Adum* (Adum son of Ojo), and that it lived upstream near the markets of Oguta. The cult of *Ojoye Adum* was a private affair. As time went bye, the spirit's reputation grew both in the village and amongst neighbors. The spirit began to make more grandiose claims for itself. It claimed to have moved down from Gout area and that it has taken charge of some of the local waters formerly under the guardianship of *Domineer*. Perhaps, the Orusangama people resented being junior partners in the cult of *Duminea* and perhaps they welcomed the chance to achieve exclusive spiritual control over their territorial waters, Orusangama people firmly adopted *Ojoye Adum* as the spirit in charge of, at least, part of their territorial waters and made him the custodian of the fish and shell fish that were the main sources of the people's subsistence. At this time, Orunagama began to experience new economic development. The shell Petroleum Company came to prospect for oil; this entailed getting labour, unskilled young men from the community were recruited into the labor force. Wages were attractive and young men abandoned fishing for Shell work. Young women frequently abandoned their fishermen husbands in favour of the newly rich wage earners.

It was in the heat of all these that *Ojoye Adum* told the community that he was the custodian of the resources below the waters. He then requested constant festivities at his shrine, in order to facilitate the striking of oil. The community agreed to this demand and accorded to him the new portfolio of Petroleum Resources and Extraction. As the company drilled deeper and deeper without striking oil, worried representatives of the community consulted *Ojoye Adum*, who admitted responsibility. The deity was angry with the Shell Petroleum Company who did not first consult and beg the water spirit that owned it. Consequently, he had "drawn" the oil out of the way of the drilling bit and would continue to do so until his stipulated conditions had been fulfilled. These included the sacrifice of several rams. A delegation was sent to the Shell Petroleum Company to explain the situation and solicit financial aid for the sacrifice. However, it was refused. The drilling continued, still with no success. Finally, rumors began to spread that the Shell Petroleum Company would soon abandon the site as a failure and move out. In desperation, the community mobilized its own finances for the sacrifices.

Soon afterwards, the Shell Petroleum Company Struck oil and *Adum's* claims were regarded as vindicated. However, the community's prosperity declined and gradually the cult of the deity dwindled. Moreover, the chief priest of the cult got himself into a series of problem, some of them stemming from his propensity for making improper advances to clients and to villagers' wives. Before long he died, and the diagnosis was that *Adum* killed him for persistently infringing his laws. With the death of the medium and priest of the deity, the cult fell into neglect. People began to rely once more on *Duminea* for the regularity of their harvests of fish and shellfish. This story exemplifies the process for adopting a new god.

It has also been observed that the traditional religious concepts of a heavenly being with creative powers among the Zulus of South Africa, known as *Unkulunkulu*, has undergone a change in the sense that Christianity has adopted that name for God (Sundkler 1961: 370). Also, a significant development in the therapeutic system of the herbalist has taken place too. The case of the herbalist *Nyanga* is a typical example. The *Nyanga* treat hysteria with medicines meant to replace the hysteria with some form of possession. The "Zionist" prophet movement, strongly opposed these practices, instead the Zionist claim that they are able to cure or replace the possession induced by the *Nyanga*, with the possession of the Holy Spirit. As a result the Zionist churches created a syncretistic system of purification rites, taboos, faith healing and witch hunting. This syncretism led to the development of a church centered on the purification rites in the sacred pond. The Zionist prophets have formed a modern movement of witch-finders that, in many ways, have replaced the "heathen" witch-finders. The existing "heathen" patterns of divination were closely approximated by this new movement, with some modifications to suit modern conditions.

Modern changes could be seen in the traditional religions practiced in most parts of Africa. According to Horton (1988) the Yoruba god, *Ogun,* by the beginning of this century had as its portfolio, the production and use of iron. Believed to have lived a brave and adventurous life on earth *Ogun* became the founder of new settlements. In the spiritual realm, he is believed to bestow his personal attributes and qualities on his votaries, mainly hunters and blacksmiths. In modern Yorubaland, *Ogun* is still viewed as the spiritual guiding force for hunters and blacksmiths, and is now the patron deity of people in the iron making and iron using industry, such as car drivers, mechanics and engineers, rail-workers, security men and those in the armed forces. Other people not in the above category take to *Ogun* with the belief that he will deliver them from car accidents and military coups. As a result of the experience of slavery, oppression and dehumanization, *Ogun* took up the portfolio of "Leader of Revolution" in Brazil.

As has been shown above, African religious and cultural institutions are die-hards. The African cosmology is adaptive, changing according to changing circumstance and times. Therefore, as already mentioned, for any model to adequately explain the uniqueness of the nature of change found in Africa, it must duly recognize the ambivalent elements of change and continuity.

Chapter Three: The Emu People

3.0 Geographical Location

Emu is one of the six clans in Ndokwa West Local Government Area of Delta State. It is about 100 kilometers from Asaba, the capital of the state; 200 kilometers from Benin and about 60 Kilometers from Warri. The town is situated between latitude 5°38-4°2N and longitude 6°13-6°25E of the Greenwich Meridian. The clan shares boundaries with Utagba-Ogbe (Kwale) on the North; Ozoro on the South; Abbi on the West; Ogune on the Southwest and Ashaka on the East. Its land area is approximately 44 square Kilometers and spans about 36 kilometers along Abraka/Kwale Road. The clan with annual rainfall of about one meter lies mainly in the flat rain forest belt of Niger Delta and less than 100 meters above the sea level. The climate is humid with mild temperature in the two distinct rainy and dry seasons. Demographically, its population numbering about 150, 000, ranks amongst the highest in the local government area. The 1973 national census placed Emu as the ninth most densely populated community in the Ndokwa region.

3.1 The Origin of the People

The Emu community was one of the off-shoots of the latest Eastern and Western Igbo settlements at the end of the seventeenth and early eighteenth century respectively. There have been diverse versions of locally circulated stories concerning the origin of the Emu people. One of the versions holds that, the founder of this clan was a man called *Olor*. *Olor* and his wife, Emu, migrated from Onitcha-Ukwuani presumably following an alleged homicide that *Olor* committed. As the couple fled, they took with them the *Ofo* (the household god). The *Ofo* is of a great religious importance amongst the Igbo and it is always in the custody of the heir of the family of clan. The heir is the eldest son of the family. The Onitcha-Ukwuani people, who were very incensed by the disappearance of the Ofo, went after Olor and his wife to recover their god. *Olor* and *Emu*, in escape, crossed the river on a mysterious log. The log was later identified as an alligator. This miraculous escape that was wrought by the alligator made alligator the totem animal of Emu people.

The name of their settlement after their escape was *Emu*; it was derived from the name of Olor's wife. They had two sons named *Ikosa* and *Ebilige*. While they were in Emu, some other people migrated from Isoko and Ndoshimili to join them. These were the Ogbolum family from Emevor in Isokoland and Umuodio family from Akarai in Ndoshimili. With a population explosion in their original settlement, Emu expanded its territory, thereby founding newer territories such as *Emu-Obi-Ogo*; *Emu-Obodeti*; *Emu-Ebendo*; *Ekpu-Ikpe* and *Iyasele*. The last two later integrated to form *Emu-Iyasele* (Ogolime, oral interview).

Another version of the origin of the Emu people posits that they migrated from Benin kingdom to settle in the place they are found today. According to this version, the man called *Olor* who founded Emu, had a wife called *Emu*, after whom the settlement was named. They came from Benin and encountered a big river with no means of crossing. It is said that an alligator, known as *Onyemu*, aided their crossing. Today, *Onyemu* is a sacred animal in Emu because of the help it rendered to the founders of Emu. Upon crossing over from Onitcha Ukwuani, Olor and his wife settled at one end of the town. There they encountered Itimi people and there was a great war between them. In this clash, they killed many of Itimi people. Thence they relocated to the present location of Emu. The initial place of settlement was converted into a cemetery because of the people they had killed. And until date, that area remains a sort of evil forest. It is further held by this version that in the course of dwelling in this new place other people came to join *Olor* and his wife. *Olor* had many children. These children decided that they should acquire more lands. One of the children named *Obiogoti*, allegedly left Emu, to found *Emu-Obiogo*. Another of Olor's sons *Obodoetiti* went away to establish *Emu-Obodoeti*. Then the son named *Ebendindo* founded *Emu-Ebendo* and finally the one called *Iyasele*, founded *Emu-Iyasele*. This last one shares boundary with Ashaka, a neighboring village (Ogolime, 2001).

In yet another version recounted by Egwueneu Adamgbodomgbo, the father of Ezemu migrated with his children-*Ezeti*, *Ezeodu*, *Ezemu* and *Isulamani*, from Onitcha-Olona to Utagba-Uno. *Ezeodu*, *Ezemu* and *Isulamani* abandoned their ancestral settlement at Umuseti and were absorbed by other Onicha group settlers. *Isulamani*, the youngest, was integrated with Ojogwu's settlement in Isumpe-Awameka. *Ezeodu* and

Ezemu joined Emu and Onitcha-Ukwuani respectively (Staff of Office 1999: 19). *Emu*, son of Ezemu, however, was a hunter and his occupation drove him far from Amorji village of Onitcha-Ukwuani into the forest bordering Ozoro and Ilue-Ologbo in Isokoland. This new settlement later was named after him as Emu (Staff of Office 1999: 19).

The heterogeneity of the clans in Ndokwa has led to the different views held with regards to the historical origin of the people. The general opinion from among the various historians of the clan is that Emu people were the product of three major waves of migration. There were, however, other migrations that followed these major movements of people into Ndokwaland. According to our oral source, Ogolime (2001), the first wave of migration settlements included Akashaida, Ebendi and Akarai clans, who allegedly migrated from Benin. The second set of immigrants included Umu-Barautchi, Ndoni, Onyia and Adiai people, the people settled along the bank of River Niger. They were the initial group of Igbo settlers to come to Ndokwa and establish clans. It is important to note that these clans are today located in Rivers state. The third wave of migration came from an organized expedition from Edo by the end of the 7th century. These settlements included Aboh, Abbi, Amai, Umukwata and Orogum. There were in addition to these, independent Edo settlements, which included Ase, Okpai, and Ibedini. Subsequently, there were more migrations which gave rise to mixed Eastern and Western settlements of the clans of Utagba, Onitcha, Akoku, Emu, Umuolu and Umutu. Onyia also has a mixed Igbo and Ijaw immigrants (Ogolime, 2001).

3.2 Emu Worldview

The worldview of a people has been summed up as the complex of their beliefs and attitudes concerning the origin, the nature, structures, organization and interaction of beings in the universe with particular reference to humans (Ikenga-Metuh, 1987: 48). In addition to a multiplicity of beings, concepts, and attitudes which they share, religion is the underlying logic which holds them together (Ikenga-Metuh 1987: 61). Emu worldview divides the world into two, the visible and the invisible. The visible world consists of mankind and all things they can see, their visible environment, the sky, earth, forest, mountains and so forth. The invisible world consists of the heavenly realm which is located in the sky and is the home of the creator and deities. The spirit-land is the home of the ancestors/ancestresses, while the spirits and disembodied spirits are located somewhere inside the ground. However, these two worlds are not parallel; they are overlapped.

The Emu people, like every other Igbo group, subscribe to the existence of five categories of spiritual beings. These are the Supreme Being (*Chukwu*), the deities (*Mmuo*), the spirit-forces (*Alusi*), and the ancestors/ancestresses (*Nde-Iche/Umuada*) and medicine (*Ogwu*). Chukwu, the Supreme Being, is the great source of being, who brought other spirits into existence to serve his purposes. These spiritual beings are acknowledged and worshipped in honour of the Supreme Being. There are many homes which have shrines dedicated to *Chi*, the guardian angel. In these homes, God's invoked daily during morning prayers. The family head or the officiating priest in the household breaks kola-nut and calls *Chukwu* to come and eat kola-nut.

The position of the Supreme Being as a creator and giver of life is shown in the various names and attributes used to address him. He is *Chukwu-Okike* (the creator of life); *Chukwu-ma-*(God know all things); *Ifeanyi-chukwu* (nothing is too difficult for God) and so forth. The belief in deities (*Mmuo*) and spirits (*Alusi*) seems to occupy their daily attention. These deities and spirits can bless people, when a proper harmony is maintained and at the same time punish people when this harmony is disrupted. Most of these deities and spirit forces are associated with natural phenomena such as the sky, earth, rivers, and animals, etc. Some of these divinities are *Olonemu* (the ancestor divinity), *Nze* (the god of war and security), *Ani* (the earth divinity), *Igba* (patron divinity of iron), *Ossai* (the patron god of children), *Ikenga* (the god of power and success), *Odemode* (fertility god), and *Umuada* (god of fidelity).

3.3 Olonemu

Olor is the river deity or river-goddess. According to Emu mythology *Ezemu* (father of Olor) brought a shrine of a rivers goddess from Onitcha-Olona and installed it in his house for the protection of his family. Another version of the story suggested that *Olor* was an incarnate of a river-goddess, whose shrine was installed at the side of *Mgbugbu-aka*, a brook near Ogbe-Elishi quarter of Amorji in Onitcha-Ukwuani. The divinity *Olonemu* is a fusion of three gods: *Olor*, *Emu* and *Nze* (comparable to Christian trinity). *Olor* and *Emu* are male and female gods (husband and wife, deified after their death). *Nze* is the symbolic ancestral god of Umu-Onitcha, which by inheritance, followed Emu from Umu-Onicha. The fusion of theses gods explains why *Nze* has no special shrine in each family, unlike what is obtainable to Umu-Onitcha quarters or family descendants of Umu-Onticha in Utagba-Uno.

It was from Umu-Onicha on his journey to Emu that *Olor* moved his shrine to his new abode. Coincidentally, the people of Amorji still serve *mgbugbu-Aka* just as Emu people still serve *Olor* in the brook *(Edu-Olor)*. The shrine of *Olor* is situated at a brook called *Edu,* west of their settlement. When the founders of Emus found this brook, they named it *Olor,* they named that it bears till date. *Olor* and *Emu* dug and buried a part of the shrine at a spot by the side of brook. They took the other part to be installed in their settlement, perhaps, that it may serve as an alternate shrine in the event they lose the parcel of land at the brook. The content of the shrine that was buried at the brook was not revealed to their children\descendants.

The taboo of *Olonemu* is that her children (the Emu People) should not kill or watch the killing of an alligator (*Oba, Nne-Emu, and Nnem Onicha*). They should not kill or watch the killing of a ram (*Ebunu*). In the cases of the alligator, it is completely forbidden to eat the flesh of it. Emu people should regard and tread it as their "mother" (*Nne-Emu* or *Nne-Onicha*). The alligator is to be mourned and buried with reverence whenever it is found dead. It is said in Emu folklore that, several of these alligators formed a mysterious log/raft with their backs which Emu people used to cross a rivers during their migration. Of importance is that Emu, Umu-Onicha and Ndoni forbid the alligator for the same reason. It is also important to note that the *Nze* of Emu and that of Umu-Onicha have the same sanctions and prohibitions. The Emu People call it *Nne-Emu* while Onicha people call it *Nnem Onicha* (Elegbute, 2003).

3.4 Nze

Nze amongst the Emu people is known as the god of war and the custodian of mental health. A legend holds that there was a certain monster (mermaid) called *Odogwu* that terrorized and killed the Aboh people. This monster lived in a river that was between Aboh and Isala. One day, the people of Aboh consulted a diviner, who told them to go to a village called Odo-egiliga and inquire of a leper known as Obumkpumkpu. They were told that it was only this leper that had a solution to their problem and can assist them in killing the mermaid. The people of Aboh did as they were directed but did not meet Obumkpumkpu. They however, met his mother, Ikpenyi, who helped to fetch her son. Upon discussing with the Aboh people, they agreed to fight the monster on *Eke-Uku* day. The following items were needed for the fight: a day old baby, a black dog, a chicken, a piece of white cloth, and a red skirt (*Mbenuku*).

On the appointed day, Obumkpumkpu got to Aboh and requested for a canoe with two strong men to paddle it. With these two men; he went to the river in search of the monster. Soon the monster appeared near the canoe and attempted to capsize the canoe. Obumkpumkpu picked up the one day old baby and showed it to the monster. This neutralized the powers of the monster, and the monster placed its head on the edge of the canoe as if asleep. Obumkpumkpu threw the chicken into the river and proceeded to cut off the head of the monster. Being a leper and without fingers it was a very tedious job for him. When Obumkpumkpu finally cut off the head of the monster, the body of the monster sank into the river while the head fell into the canoe. The people of Aboh cut off the jaw of the monster and gave it to Obumkpumkpu. However, Obumkpumkpu charged the people of Aboh to keep their own part of the head and to make a shrine for it. They were to worship it as their god of war. He also told them what the prohibitions of this god were and how to venerate it. The Emu people and Aboh have the *Nze* for the same purpose.

On returning from his mission at Aboh, Obumkpumkpu was exiled from his village. He traveled through Emu-Ebendo to Emu-Obodeti with his escort. He finally came to his family in Emu-Unor, where his father, Iyasele, received him. Iyasele asked his friend Ogbolum to take Obumkpumkpu who refused to enter the house insisting that the bag he had on him will not enter into anyone's house. A hut had to be erected outside Ogbolum's house for his friend's son to keep his bag. Obumkpumkpu kept the bag and the machete (*Ogbodo*) with which he cut off the monster's head in the hut. He later called Ogbolum and showed him the contents of the bag and also told him how he got it. He called it *Nze*, a god of war. He went on to explain the prohibitions of this god and also how to serve it. Thus, Ogbolum assumed the position of the priest of *Nze* (*Oyiwa*) in Emu.

Nze is worshipped with a ram that is neither killed nor harmed. When the priest presents the ram to the divinity, the white cloth of *Nze* is tied around the neck of the ram and it is left to roam about in the village, until it dies on its own. Any ram used in the worship of *Nze* belongs to *Nze* and it is called *Ebunu-Nze*. It becomes a sacred animal and everyone in the village treats the ram with reverence. The following are the prohibitions of Nze:

1. The adherents shall not have sex with a female slave.
2. They shall not kill a ram or watch it killed, but they may eat its meat, only if it is killed by a non-native. (Enuademu, 2003)

3.5 Ani

This god and its worship came to Emu through its founder. According to Emu folklore: when Olor arrived at Emu, he planted an Iroko tree and called it *Ani*. He began to worship it. The tree was meant to symbolize the ownership of the land on which the tree is. It is therefore known as the earth divinity in charge of landed properties. There are several taboos to this god. Strict adherence to these taboos is demanded from the people. Most especially, the divinity has stipulated sacred days. On these days, most social and economic activities are prohibited. All forms of disobedience are visited with varied sanctions, but all geared towards appeasing *Ani*. For instance, it is a taboo to go to the farm on sacred days and anyone that does so has to appease *Ani* with a sacrifice. The sacrifice is done after planting and staking of yams in a new farming season.

Ani forbids the death of a pregnant woman. If this happens, it is assumed that the divinity is not pleased and as such nobody is expected to go to the farm, break palm kernel, cut firewood, or play music for nine days. After the period of nine days, the family of the deceased woman would buy a ram, ten tubers of yam, a piece of white cloth, and a keg of palm wine. These are offered as sacrifice to cleanse the land. The sacrifice is followed by singing in front of *Ani* at the centre of the town. Nobody goes to the farm that day. Normal activities resume only after these observances (Elegbute, 2003).

3.6 Ossai

It is the people's belief that the deity *Ossai* came from Isokoland. This is the god of fertility to Emu people, so, anyone seeking children consorts with *Ossai*. Thus, *Ossai* is a personal god, each family owns and keeps a shrine for it within their compound. One of the rites that must be performed by the worshippers is sacrifice of a rooster to Ossai by the husband of woman that births a child. If he fails to do this at the time of the birth of the child, the child will fall sick. However, this god can be appeased by an immediate sacrifice of a cock by the father of the child (Enyabegwu, 2003).

3.7 Odede

Odede is sometimes referred to as the god of sex or the fertility god. This god, which was allegedly founded and instituted by a man, regulates the activities associated with the menstrual cycle of a woman. Odede has so many prohibitions among which are that no one was to have sex in a farm. During menstruation, women are not to go to the farm; a woman whose period starts while in the farm must leave the farm immediately, and no man should have sex with a woman during menstruation. There are however, exceptions to some of these rules, especially for those that live in the outskirts of the town. The elders in these outskirts offer as sacrifice to Odede a cock and plant an iroko tree in each of the various hamlets. With this sacrifice, they proclaim that their residence is not on the farm in spite of the location of their homes, consequently, they will be free to have sex in their houses.

3.8 Ikenga

Ikenga is the god of power and success. In times of danger, it gives guidance to the people; it protects from injuries, particularly during the farming period. At the end of each farming season, the people offer sacrifices to *Ikenga* to express their gratitude for this protection. This deity is involved in the coronation of a chief, as gratitude, the person that gets the chieftancy title, makes an offering of a goat (Enyabegwu, 2003).

3.9 Olokoto

Olokoto is the patron divinity of commerce. This deity was initiated and institutionalized by very strong and brave women. The names of these prominent women are *Ikpe* and *Ashaba*. Olokoto is served by the entire community whenever there is an economic recession. For this, a goat and a hen are sacrificed to appease the god (Enyabegwu, 2003).

3.10 Igba

The *Igba* deity is the god of war and the patron divinity of iron. The belief is that offers protection to the people in times of war. To obtain this security, the people drink water obtained from inside the shrine. The drunk water will render the body of the user impervious to machete and bullet. The priest of this god is called *Eze-Igba*. When one is appointed into this priesthood, he kills a goat before his confirmation. If he cannot afford the goat, the position would be given to another person. There are numerous taboos and prohibitions surrounding the worship of *Igba*. None should eat snails or a fused plantain; women during the menstrual period should not walk pass through the shrine; and men and women do not enter the shrine after they have had sexual intercourse. There are however a few exceptions to these rules. The person that eats the forbidden foods (such as snail, and/or fused-plantains) begins to spit uncontrollably. Sacrifices are then offered to appease *Igba* and the person will be healed (Enuademu, 2003).

3.11 Umuada

An *ada* is the eldest woman among the women in the Emu community and she is the custodian of the god that binds all women in their marriages. This god is known as *Umuada*. It can also be said to be a god of fidelity or feminine purity. Sexual infidelity or extramarital sex is prohibited. Hence, if a woman commits adultery, and fails to confess to it, her children will continue to die, one after the other, until she confesses. If she admits to committing the adultery, she would go to the *Ada* who would offer a sacrifice on her behalf. She would be made to confess all her unfaithfulness before the shrine. She will thereafter kill a goat and then be made free. Where she fails to admit to her acts, the whole cycle of the affliction of the god will resume, until total confession is made. The deity is concerned with minor issues such as another man discussing sex with a married woman and she fails to tell her husband. After some time, the god will strike the woman with an illness which can only be abated by a sacrifice to the god (Idonor Isakpa 1990).

3.12 Nde-Iche

Nde-Iche deity is of ancestral origin. The *Nde-Iche* are the founders and guardians of traditional laws and customs as well as morality. It is thus a personal god that is found in every family. Each family has its own shrine. Formerly, this god had only one shrine where people go to offer sacrifices. This main shrine was at Ikosa region of the Emu community. The town of Ebilije later set up its own shrine. There are no clear cut prohibitions attributed to this deity, but if an Emu person commits any evil against the laws of the land, this god will afflict such a person with irregular breathing by stopping the inter-coastal muscles from relaxing. This sickness makes it clear, that the person is afflicted by *Nde-Iche*.

Apart from the ancestors (*Nde-Iche*) who form the category of human spirits, there also are the wandering spirits of evil men and women who lived and died unwholesome death. These evil spirits, presumed not to have reached the spirit land of the ancestors, constitute the sources of suffering and misfortune to Emu people. Hence, the people strive to manipulate benevolent forces to assuage these evil forces in order to achieve good living. How a man achieves this task depends on his ability to woo the benevolent forces to keep in check the works of the malevolent ones (Udechukwu in Kalu, 1978: 87). Emu people, like their Igbo neighbors, believe that for them to maintain a harmonious relationship with all these categories of spiritual beings, they must keep in touch with the spiritual world through divination, intersectional prayers, and above all engaging the services of the *dibie* or medicine men, to fortify them with ritual medicines.

3.13 Political Structure of the Emu People

In Emu, family and kinship system are the basic social units. Emu upholds a localized patrilineal system (*Umu-Nnadi*). The lineage bears the name of the presumed founding father. Lineage varies in size according to the number of male offspring in the ancestral lineage. Emu, the ancestral founder of Emu clan, had two sons, Ebilije and Umukofuni (Ikosa). Ebilije begot Onodi, Odigwe-Ejine, Okopala-Ogba, and Useh Ojech. These people constitute the major ancestral family units in the line of Ebilije. Umukofuni begot Ikosa Ajanogu, Almona, Oka and Iyesele, the major ancestral family units in the line of Umukofuni. Ikosa-Okpi is an extension of Ikosa Uku in the group of Umukofuni. These ancestral fathers are the founder of the six villages of Emu namely: Ebilije, Umukofuni, Emu-Obiogo, Emu-Obodeti, Emu-Ebendo and Emu-Iyasele. The *Ogbe* constitutes the major ancestral family unit in Emu (Ogolime, 2001).

Major family units contain segments of closely related family groups (*Ebo*) that live together in places where their forefathers had lived. Within the *Ebo* are clusters of more closely related family units (*Imusu*), they also live together in places where their forefathers had resided. The *Imusu* are families of persons of one father, a household unit, which is the nucleus of the localized patrilineal *Umu-Nnadi* (children of one ancestral father). The main characteristics of the household include allegiance to a common ancestral father, maintaining one shrine (*Nde-iche*), having one totem animal, observing a common law of progeny and practicing exogamy.

Women occupy two positions within the family unit. A woman has a position within her patrilineal home and within her husband's home. Though assimilated into her husband's family, a married woman may return to her father's family to become the *Ada* of her father's village. The *Ada* is the oldest female person in the village. By her status, the *Ada* is the high priestess of the goddess of feminine purity (*Umu-Ada*) and is greatly respected by all women in the village. The custom allows a widow to retain her full membership status in the family of the late husband and is entitled to allocation of the family farmlands, for the up-keep of her children, as long as she does not remarry. Her right to such land derives from her children by virtue of their patrilineal descent.

The government of Emu is formerly vested in the *Okpala-Uku*-in-Council; this was made up of the *Okpala-Uku,* the *Okwa* and the *Inotu*. With the recent introduction of the institution of kingship, the government shifted from the *Okpala-Uku*-in-Council to the king and his council of chiefs, known as the *Ezemu*-in-Council. The first monarch, that is, the 1st *Ezemu* of Emu Kingdom hailed from Umu-Afonta Royal Family in Amoji Village of Onicha Ukwuani. This *Ezemu* reigned for fifty-five years (1545–1600). Agbadu reigned as the 2nd *Ezemu* for twelve years (1600–1612). His son, Ugbo at the age of thirty-seven ascended the throne and reigned for sixteen years (1612–1628). He was assassinated by his subjects. It was Okpala-Ogbodo of Ikosa, who at about 1711 evolved an administrative system based on age grade, and consequently, gerontocracy emanated. This evolution caused a vacuum in the royal administration for eighty three years (Staff of Office 1999: 9–21).

Emu's form of gerontocracy consists in an *Okpalas* who has absolute spiritual and temporal powers and exercises control over the people of their villages. Each *Opkala* is subject to the most senior person in their *Okpala* age group (the *Okpala-Uku*-in-Council). Thus, in the interregnum, the *Okpala-Uku*-in-Council and the *Okpala*-in-Council ruled Emu from the beginning of the nineteenth century (1806) to the time of the coronation of king Ulu, the fourth Ezemu of Emu kingdom on 5th April, 1999 (Staff Office 1999: 22). This coronation marked the end of gerontocracy, the restoration of the monarchy, and the revival of kingship rule in Emu. Emu people are formally arranged in a hierarchical order based on age group within the society. The age grades are represented in the table below:

➢ The king	
➢ *Okpala Ukwu*	above 80 years
➢ *Okwa*	80 years
➢ *Ivulawai*	70 years
➢ *Inotu*	50 years
➢ *Otuole*	40 years
➢ *Otu Onu Ogba*	30 years
➢ *Otu Nkpulaku*	23 years
➢ *Otu Aya*	17 years

Within the above societal configuration, the people graduate from one age group to another starting from the bottom of the social pyramid.

3.14 Social life and Calendar of Festivities

The social life in Emu is punctuated includes various festivals that are observed at specific intervals during the year. Festivities are held in February, June, November, and December. Prominent among the festivals are the *Ukwuata, Ikenge* and *Ime Eze Emu*.

3.14.1 Ukwuata Festival

There are several different views as to the origin of the *Ukwuata* festival. Some believe that it originated from *Eziokpor*, a village in *Umu-Akashiade* group of *Ukwuani*. In some other quarters, it is said to have originated from Abbi, a town located three Kilometres west of Emu. Other people emphasize the common ancestral link and cultural similarities with *Etua* in *Onicha-Ukwuani* in order to claim that *Ukwuata* festival originated there. *Ukwuata* is a socio-religious festival, which occurs before the beginning of a new farming season in Emu. The festival commences on any *Eke-Uku* market day as may be designated, between the end of January and third week of February every year. It lasts for about fifteen days. It is accompanied by lots of feasting in every home. During the festivity people are prohibited from going to the farm and from fighting. Violation of these rules attracts heavy penalties.

There are social and religious aspects to *Ukwuata* festival. The social aspect begins with *Agha Ukwuata* on *Afor* market day which is the seventh day of the proclamation of the festival by the *Okpala-Uku* in collaboration with the *Okwas,* the *Iotus* and the *Otu-Ole* age group. Men from the two sections of the village, Ebilije and Ikosa, dance in large groups towards each other with toy-guns and wooden machetes singing native war songs and pretending to be real warriors. When the two "armies" meet and crossed each other at the centre of the village, the war ends with the song: "*Ebo baa!! Ebo naa!! ni ogwu edo!!!*" (Let everyone go! Let everyone go! The war has ended!!!)

The main *Ukwuata* attraction or activity commences on next day which is a market (*Eke*) after the mock war. A young man (*Obu Ukwuata)*, who has been selected or hired and who has learned the necessary dance steps, carries the *Ukwuata* outfit. This young man wears for this occasion special traditional clothes. With the *Ukwuata* on his head, the young performs and entertains the community. He receives applause and admiration from the spectators. The climax of the dance occurs when he performs the *Oyoyo-Obodeti Ukwuata* dance before the traditional rulers, chiefs and *Inotus* at the *Obi-ogwa*. (See Appendix 2 for a list of festivals in Emu).

The religious part of the festival begins on *Olie* market day following the social performance. The service lasts for twelve days. From the *Olie* day, the community begins to venerate the spirit of the departed ancestors, symbolized by the *Ofo* and continue to do so until the end of the worship. The main feature of these traditional rites is the compulsory homage (*Ifo Ibu*) that sons-in-law pay to their fathers-in-law. To pay this homage, a son-in-law make available following items; ten tubers of yam, sizeable mud-fish (*Mkpulu* or *Oilili*), and drinks. These items are carried by the wife to her father's family on the day that they worship their ancestor. The paying of homage continues as long as the marriage endures. It is considered a serious breach of marriage obligation if a son-in-law failed to do this annually. In place of the afore-listed items, many sons-in-law, especially those not resident in Emu send cash.

Another interesting feature of the *Ukwuata* festival is the presence of the dance group of *Olu* or *Ogonya* masquerades. The group is made up of *Ojenoku, ogbo, Ajekpe, Atu, Ikpa, Akpaha* and their leader *Echinei*, all dressed in unique costumes. This dance group performs at the end of the *Ukwuata* festival. Local history holds that at Eziokpor, one *Osele Obodagu* visited the spirit world in a trance and saw *Olu* spirits dancing. He observed their steps and when he came back from trance, he rehearsed the dance steps, then introduced them to his people (Enwemike, 2003). Another Emu folklore has it that the dance steps originated from Anyama, a riverine community along the Ase-Creek. Investigation have confirmed that the *Olu* masquerade is peculiar to the riverine people of Delta State. Hence, such appellation as *Umu-Oru* or *Nde-Olu* is used to describe the riverine people from the creeks around the River Niger (Heritage, History & culture Committee 1999: 23). The masquerades carry the designs of fish and marine colours and such animals like the alligator or crocodile. The *Eilishi-Ugbo* dance of Aboh people along the River Niger is a modified replica of the *Olu* Masquerade dance from Anyama. It depicts the dancing steps as those of the marine mermaids. It is probable therefore, that the *Olu* came from *Anyama* through *Aboh* and across *Ase*-Creeks to *Ashaka*. With Emu geographically situated further into the upland, their masquerade is often associated with the secret cult of the *Echinei* deity, whose members operate in strict seclusion. *Echinei* in Emu is a secret only to the extent that woman are forbidden to see it or enter its shrine called *Ipo*.

At the end of the *Ukwuata* festival, that is, on the fifteenth day, the *Otu-Ole* age group performs the ritual ceremony of *Ichu-Mmo*. During this ceremony, the members of this age group match through the streets of the town, bearing fire to cleanse the land of evil spirits, which they believe came to share in the festivities. With fire glowing in their hands, they match to the town's cemetery (*Amuzo*) where they make a heap of the firewood with which they chase evil spirits back to their abode in the spirit world.

3.14.2 Ikenge Festival

The *Ikenge* is an annual festival. It begins on an *Eke* day usually within the second or third week in June. It marks the end of yam planting season in Emu. Unlike *Ukwuata* festival, the *Ikenge* festival has no social connotation. It is essentially a religious festival. In the traditional sense, *Ikenge* is the god which brings good luck to people. Every adult male keeps an *Ikenge* shrine in his house and venerates it for some of the following purposes: to seek favour from ancestral spirit; to seek protection against evil spirits, particularly witches, wizards and evil minded persons; to propitiate neglected ancestral spirits or angered household deities. Besides the personal *Ikenge* shrine, there is the *Ikenge-Osa* (community *Ikenge*) that is served by the *Onotu-Ukwu* on behalf of the community for the above mentioned purpose.

The *Ikenge* festival is proclaimed by the *Okpala-Ukwu* in collaboration with the *Okpala-Uku*-in-Council and the *Otu-Ole* age group. The festival is kicked off by the *Onotu-Ukwu* on the appointed *Eke* day with the worship of *Ikenge-Osa*. This is done by the killing of a goat. This goat is cooked with yams, plantain, and special ingredients. Although this festival only last two days, there are some features of it that are worthy of note. One of them is the *Ochu* masquerade dance that is performed by men. Members of the dance group carry machetes, spears, bows and arrows. Nowadays, they are not aggressive and do not harm spectators, except when challenged or provoked. Sometimes the members of the group challenge themselves to a fight when they cross path with members of another dance group. They do this in order to test the effectiveness of the protective charms they wear.

Another important aspect of the *Ikenge* festival is the display by the *Otu Igbu*. This literally means society of killers. It is made up of all titled warriors and heroes in the clan. To qualify for membership, one must have been in a war and through bravery killed an enemy and brought back home the head or jaw of the victim as trophy. The *Igbu* society begins their activities on the second day (*Olie*) of the *Ikenge* festival (*Inwu-Olie*) with an early morning *macabre* dance. In this dance, these men, brandishing cutlasses, move from the town square to the cemetery (*Amuzo*), where they perform their ritual ceremony, known as *Iwa-Awuwa*. According to one informant, Okolugbo, war divinities and military charms which now abound in Ukwuani communities emerged as a result of Igbo raids in Emu community.

After the ceremony at the cemetery, they return to the town dancing to war songs, led by the traditional war dance troupe (*Otu Ukele*). These dances are offered as homage to the *Oyiwa*, the high priest of the war god, *Nze*. They perform some rites to *Oyiwa* that are exclusive only to initiates. Finally, they finally dance back to the house of their leader (*Odede-Igbu-u*) who keeps and serves their ritual war drum (*Okuma*) (Heritage, History & Culture Committee, 1999: 24). The *Okuma* drum is a wooden drum measuring about four feet high and two feet in diameter, it is carved out of a big tree trunk and covered at one end with human skin. *Okuma* is played in the public only during *Ikenge* festival or at the death of an initiate. This ceremony is called *Ibe Okpa* and it entails the slaying of a cock midair in front of the mock casket of the deceased. Thereafter, the drum is left in front of the casket for seven consecutive days in honour of the dead hero. The drum is returned to the *Odede-Ogbu-u* with a chicken provided by the bereaved family.

3.14.3 Ite–Otite Festival

This particular festival is basically a religious festival with several worship components. Prominent among them is the *Isume-Iji*. This is called "Roasted Yam festival" and is divided into two phases. The first is the yam roasting for elders known as *Otite Ikei*. This is performed by the *Okpala-Uku* who is the custodian of the founding father's ancestral *Ofo*. The second is known as *Otite Ebo*. Here the various family heads worship the ancestors. *Otite* consists of several newly harvested yam tubers that are roasted. These are sliced into pieces after scraping off the burnt part. Some of the burnt parts are added to a sauce made in a mortar with oil, potash, salt, roasted fish or meat and green vegetable (*okposokilike*). The vegetable is only used for *Otite*. The importance of the vegetable is reflected in the saying that, "*Alugbe Egwu Egwu te Otite*" (no child plays to the point of preparing otite soup). The dish is served to friends and relations. The male heads of families as well as the females (*Ada*) perform this ritual as a memorial worship of paternal and maternal ancestors respectively. In the evening, pounded yam is served with chicken or fish soup to relations.

3.15 Social Values

The Emu word people to describe any breach of the numerous injunctions or taboos is *Alu*. That is, abomination. Another term is *Nsu-Ani*, that is, transgressions againt the earth–god. There are, however, two classes of abominations. There are those that are related to desecration of the land and those that are morally and socially based. The following acts are seen as a desecration of the land:

1. Going to the farm on *Eke* market day:
2. Stealing yam from barns in the farm
3. Committing incest
4. Committing suicide, especially by hanging
5. Sex with a female slave or a brother's wife
6. Committing homicide
7. Poisoning someone, especially a native of Emu
8. A woman climbing a palm tree or kola-nut tree, especially if she does it with the special climbing rope, *Agbu*
9. A woman in her menstrual period going to the farm
10. Woman dying in pregnancy or during child birth or person dying in the bush/farm, all of which constitute 'bad death'

Those abominable moral and social are:

1. Adultery
2. Woman throwing their husbands onto the ground during a fight.
3. Children throwing their fathers or mother on the ground during a fight.
4. Having sex with a woman during her menstrual period.

5. Deliberately cutting off tendrils of young yam plants in another person's farm.
6. Deliberately setting another person's house or barn ablaze.
7. Disclosing the identity of the *Olu-Echinei* masquerade, especially by a woman.
8. Woman entering the *Olu-Echinei*'s shine (*ipo*) or coming out while the *Echinei* is on the routine cleansing of the house of the person who served it, or when the *Echinei* is being publicly sworn in, either by day or night;
9. Woman adorning her hair while mourning her husband, or coming out to the public within three Lunar months of the death of her husband.

Generally, a breach of any of these injunctions is a serious offence with heavy penalty. In addition to paying the penalty, the offender will be forced to provide items for rituals in order to purify the land or the household in the case of adultery committed in the house of a married person.

3.16 Economic Background

Contemporarily, Emu's economic life centers on farming, hunting, fishing, and trading. In the olden days, agriculture was the economic activity of the people. Other products and commodities needed in the community were obtained by batter. Agricultural products were exchanged for those items that were not available in the community. Farming and hunting, the traditional occupations of these people, are considered noble professions to which every man in the community aspired. Prowess and achievements were rated according to the size of one's barn or how successful a person was in his hunting expeditions. The Emu community initially was centered on the family (kindred). Production of goods was strictly meant for family consumption and excess was stored or given to the needy. Trade, as an established occupation in the community, is a recent innovation. It arose in the middle of last century, when the town expanded beyond its original borders.

The most important economic crop was the palm tree. This particular tree served the peoples' need as cash and food crop. The palm kernel was exported and or consumed locally. Also, the byproducts extracted from the tree were used for roofing, soap, and fibers. Rubber tree is a very important cash crop on the list of economic trees in Emu. This was introduced during the Second World War (1939–1945). Rubber was mainly farmed for export. The coconut tree is another important cash and food crop in the community. Its' nuts are locally consumed by the people. It was used as a means of exchange for other goods; its' demand by the neighboring communities boosted trade for Emu people. It should be noted that yam and cassava are crops still very much regarded as the principal food crops in the community. Cassava is processed into *garri* and other food items such as *Akpu*. These products are then exchanged in the market for their value. Nowadays, excess tubers of yam are sold in the market, unlike in the early times.

Chapter Four: Medicine and Medicinal Ritual in Emu

There are five fundamental elements of medicine in Emu. These fundamental elements give a clear understanding of the people's conception of medicine, what it is to them, how they use medicine and place of medicine in their lives. This chapter provides the description of these fundamental elements which include the supernatural, medicinal, taboo, spell and ritual, elements. The traditional practitioners were rarely concerned with providing definitions to their act, rather, they were more concerned with the functionality of their acts and how such improve lives in the community. The word '*Ogwu*', which literally means medicine, is also used to mean "charm" in Emu.

4.1 The Supernatural Elements of Medicine

The medicine practitioner's acts in Emu are essentially supernatural acts. The civilities of the medicine practitioner are not geared toward influencing physical laws of nature but controlling spiritual laws toward achieving certain goals. Generally, among the Igbos the power contained in medicine derives from certain patron spirit such "*agwunsi* to diviners" (Ejizu, 1989: 1380). The medicine practitioners among the Emu people obtain their powers from the water spirits. Thus, shrines of water deities (mammy water) are set up and their prohibitions are observed. Water spirits are believed to possess and guide the practitioners, who are mostly women, in dispensing prescriptions to their clients. Sometimes, the spirit of a dead ancestor/ancestress, who was a *dibie,* (medicine maker) could guide one of their children in practicing the rituals. This happens only when the living practitioner has been called into the profession by the same ancestor/ancestress who was a *dibie.*

Emu people do not consider medicine to be one of the forces of nature that can be utilized by humans, rather they regard medicine to a cherished cultural possession. To them, medicine came into the world with mankind; as such it is not something acquired by subsequent discovery in the world of nature. They strongly reject the idea of medicine as a universal impersonal power as expressed in concepts like *mana* (Pritchard, 1976: 19). The medicine practitioners do not attribute the ends of their ritual practice to their own abilities, but to a supernatural power they believe can be influenced. In their ritual practices, they make use of objects to symbolize the supernatural. The belief in the presence of the supernatural in ritual medicine is reflected in the saying among the people that: *M ge onye iwe kwa nkwa onye eka-yadi ocha ndi-iche eka nu okili kwa nkwa* (When the evil plotter beats drum for the downfall of the innocent, the gods will not let the drum sound).

4.2 The Medicinal Element of Medicine

In Emu, the term *ogwu* denotes medicine, and in a broader sense ritual preparations and charms. Comparable to Nupe people, medicine is a vernacular term applied not only to medicine and its substances but equally to medicinal herbs or drugs of any sort sourced locally or of foreign origin (i.e., from Europe), which have properties that are empirically accessible (Nadel, 1954). Medicines may be thought to have no power in themselves, or the power may be latent and only aroused through the action of a medicine man. Medicine thus become agents through which invisible beings or powers work (Parrinder, 1976: 158). Azande society considers as medicine any object in which mystical power resides and is used in ritual rites, e.g., vegetables (Evans-Pritchard, 1976: 450). Emu ritual practices combine different medicinal approaches. There are medicine rituals like *Ogwu Ashima* (medicine for premonition) and *Ogwu Ikpo Mmalu* (medicine to recall someone) that combine incantations with (herbal) medicine. This sort of medicine will work for anyone who observes the correct ceremonial processes in acquiring the medicine and one who keeps the medicine's taboos (Parrinder 1976: 158).

4.3 The Ritual Elements of Medicine

A medicinal rite could be described as goal oriented ritual performed by a lay or professional medicine practitioner according to a set procedure using herbs or animal materials. Sometimes this ritual rite may be accompanied by incantations. Some Emu medicinal rites require no rigid, fixed or set formulaic procedures to be followed scrupulously in order to attain a certain result. Important in Emu medicinal rites is adherence to the proper procedure in the admixture of the medicinal ingredients and the observances of the rites that activates the potency of the medicinal components. Generally, incantations recited during rituals are more of an informal address meant to give power and direction to the power inherent in the medicine. The emotional settings, gestures, and expressions of the medicine man during ritual performances are sometimes imitative as in *Ogwu Ifemmili* (medicine to ward off rainfall) and *Ogwu Ikpo Mmalu* (medicine to recall someone). However, imitative magic is not always present in all rites, they are absent in *Ogwu Iwa Ugboko* (medicine of command in the forest). Thus, the efficacy of the rites does not lie primarily in the ritual performance. These rites are symbolic representation of an idea or belief that are expressed during the process of influencing the supernatural to a certain goal.

4.4 The Spell Elements of Medicine

A spell is the spoken word believed to have supernatural powers when recited during medicinal rituals. This spell or incantation may be recited for positive or negative ends as in *Ogwu ashima* (medicine for premonition) and *Ogwu Ibo Mmalu Onu* (medicine of curse). The spell may begin with a form of adoration and ends with a request or command. A spell could be whispered or spoken aloud during the medicinal ritual. In Emu, similar to Azande ritual practices, the mediciner addresses the medicines and tells them what he wants them to do. The mediciner is free to with how they utter the incantations, this is unlike the Yoruba incantations, where the reciter must adhere to a prescribed form of utterance, using the right words and correct sentences; a minor variation of the wordings may render the incantation useless. The Emu medicinal spell similar to Buyoro serves to activate the power that resides in the medicine. "This activation requires a form of words or a spell. The medicine is addressed informally or more rarely, in a set phrase" Beattie (1963: 37).

4.5 The "Taboo" Elements of Medicine

A ritual taboo is an important element in the successful performance of medicinal rites in Emu. In Emu the medicine practitioners are hedged round by taboos; they must refrain from eating certain foods, from causal sexual indulgence and from many prescribed contaminating actions. Unless the medicine practitioners rigidly observe these taboos their charms will lose their potency. However, in Emu it is not in all ritual performances that the medicine practitioner would have to observe taboos. Some ritual medicines such as *Ogwu Iwa Ugboko* (medicine of command in the forest) retain their potency irrespective of the medicine practitioner's ritual behaviour. For the Emu people, an infraction on ritual prohibition would at worst only bring about a negation of the goals of such medicinal performance. It is believed that before a ritual is carried out, there must be a purpose or goal which the ritual is aimed at achieving. Hence, the Emu saying that, *Ugo e je afia ni nkiti* (an eagle does not go to the market place unless there is something there). There are many purposes to which a medicinal ritual could be sought, the most of these are personal and communal welfare, protection from the evil intention of others, and for vengeance.

4.6 Witchcraft and Sorcery

In scholarly discourse, distinction is made between medicine, witchcraft, sorcery and divination, but not all scholars accept this differentiation. According to Dopamu (1979: 14), the notion that Africans do not distinguish between witchcraft and evil medicine may be true of some African people, but it is erroneous to generalize such conceptions across Africa. Where these distinctions do not occur, the concepts are used interchangeably, thus creating a certain amount of confusion. In many African localities, different words are used for witchcraft and sorcery each of the terms. Witchcraft is seen as a bad medicine directed to cause the destruction of other people. Witchcraft is characterized by the lack of any palpable apparatus connected with it; there are no rites, ceremonies, incantations, or invocations, the force is projected at will from the mind of the witch (Olusakin, 2014: 138). Sorcery is bad magic. It is the art of attaining objectives, acquiring knowledge, and performing works of wonders through supernatural or non-rational means (Ellwood, 2008: 1). Its aim is to destroy, kill, maim and jeopardize the wellbeing of the society. It is destructive medicine made through the manipulation of the cosmic order (Owete and Iheanacho, 2009: 145). The techniques used in these medicines are similar to those used in good magic. They include chants, spells, gestures or actions. So, it is antisocial.

According to Alana (2000: 210) sorcery is practiced in various ways. A type works through contact; its' victim can be harmed by initiating contact with anything that had touched the victim's body such as the victim's nails, spittle, urine, sweat, clothes, and even footprint. These objects can be spiritually manipulated to harm the person (contagious medicine). Contagious sorcery also works through burial of charms in the ground (Owete and Iheanacho 2009: 145). Another type of sorcery works through space. Space or distance is not a barrier to this type of sorcery. The target may "be invoked to appear in shape and figure in a ritual mirror and is spiritually infested or attacked with harmful medicine" (Owete and Iheanacho, 2009: 146). Also, the soul of the person can be pinned down with pegs or a clay image made of his body and thorns stuck into the vital organ. The enemy will then feel the pain in those spots and may die (Parrinder 1954: 117). The target can only escape such attack if he/she possesses a higher power (Alana 2000: 210). The third type works through confrontation. The intended victim has to be physically present so as to hear the evil incantations that will generate an intended harm.

Calling down lightning upon a victim is another type of sorcery so also is the poisoning of a target's food or drinking water. Magical powder may also be secretly poured around a target's premises. Sorcerers are said to have animal familiar working for them. Thus, they can transform themselves into a choice animal-familiar such as snake, bird, or leopard, in order to cause havoc. They can also use dead bodies or semi animal familiars; these are small hairy beings, often with only one leg, and they could make a demonic gnome and place it on the victims' premises or at crossroads (Parrinder 1954: 119).

Witchcraft and sorcery ae believed to share certain relationship. Hence, some societies and scholars do not see any difference between them, but to some, the two have areas of divergence. This may be because; the old English word "Wicca" from which the word witch derived is also used to describe a person who practices magic. So also the Greek root pharmakos from which the English pharmacy was coined. Pharmakos refers to drugs, potions and poison. The root word of the concepts translates to sorcery, sorcerer, and witchcraft (K. A. Kitchen, 1962: 723). Besides, both witches and sorcerers tend toward the same end; they are workers of evil. The Yoruba for example, though recognize the difference between the two; still group them together with all evildoers. All of them are given the general name *aye* (the world). The world, in this context, is the concentration of the powers of evil (Idowu, 1991: 173). Also, Mbiti (1975: 165) sees evil magic as forces in the hand of certain individuals, while witchcraft is the force in manifestation which may be in–born, inherited or acquired. Parrinder (1954: 123) however records that even the societies that see the two as one, still believe they have areas of divergence. Parrinder prefers to use 'day witches' for sorcerers and 'night witches' for witches. For Alana (2002: 209), the two are not the same. The one who practices witchcraft (witch) is called *aje* among the Yoruba, while a sorcerer is *Oso* or *Ologun Ika* (the one with wicked charms).

Sorcerers are mainly men, while witches are mainly women. Sorcerers make use of magical apparatus to achieve their aim, while witches use inherent psychic power. Sorcery is acquired through learning and apprenticeship, while witchcraft is acquired through food or spiritual transfer. All sorcerers are conscious of their activities, some witches may not be aware of their actions. Sorcerers do not have council or guild, though two or more of them can come together to harm a common enemy, witches normally have guilds. The activities of sorcerers are physical, while the activities of witches are spiritual. Sorcerers carry out their wicked acts both day and night, witches' activities are carried out at night. Sorcerers do not eat their victims; witches eat theirs in the spirit. Sorcerers could be approached to purchase bad magic, since witches are not known, they have no clients. Lastly, while sorcery is totally evil, witchcraft may be used for the protection of loved ones (Alana, 2000: 213–214).

In Emu community, witchcraft is not an observable phenomenon like the sorcerer's bad medicine.

> When I speak of witchcraft, I refer to that, which is real, and that affects the life of Africans in every walk of life; witchcraft is an urgent and very harassed reality. This means that whatever may be our own theories or preconceived notions about witchcraft, we can only help the African if we sit where he sits try and see the thing in his own light, and get to the rest of his belief in such a diabolic, soul-enslaving influence (Idowu (1975: 46).

What Idowu says of witchcraft accurately describes Emu people's beliefs. According to Pritchard (1966: 387) "...the difference between a sorcerer and a witch is that the former uses the technique of medicine and derives his power from medicine, while the later acts without rites and spells. He uses psycho-psychical powers to achieve his end". To the Emu people a sorcerer is one who practices bad ritual medicine illicitly. A medicine practitioner could be employed by the community to perform bad ritual medicine against another community or non-member of the community, in such cases, where bad ritual medicines are sanctioned by society, they are considered licit and thus acceptable.

The name for a medicine practitioner is *Dibie* with the appellation *Omenka, Ogbue bune*. The antonym to a *dibie* is the sorcerer called *dibie aju ogwu,* and a witch is known as *Ogbome*. Witchcraft among the Emu refers to innate mystical power which a possessor can use to harm other people while a sorcerer is one who is thought to practice evil medicine against others. These acts themselves are usually of such a nature that they can be performed by anyone. Among the people of Emu, a witch is one with inherent powers and innate ability which they cannot control. Consequently, witches are generally seen as agents of evil who solely perform evil acts. They are therefore seen as enemies of human society. This is why witches are hunted in Emu.

The Emu people also belief in sorcery. But unlike witches, sorcerers are not viewed as agents of evil but as people who use powers to cause harm. Unlike the witches that are not physically known except suspected, sorcerers are well known in Emu. A sorcerer manipulates spiritual laws and can cause harms by use of contagious or symbolic magic. It is believed that they could obstruct another person's progress through the manipulation of some physical materials in their possession. However, For the Emu, you can beg a sorcerer for forgiveness but you cannot beg a witch. Unlike the Azande and the Yoruba, where the sorcerer does not possess inherent malevolent power like the witch, the Emu sorcerer could possess inherent powers. These powers are not necessary malevolent but are transferable. This explains why a medicinal prescription could be given to any researcher who wants to know, but at the same time it is believed that, without the transference of the inherent medicinal powers to the acquirer, the prescription or medicine will not be effective.

4.7 Divination

There appears to be a distinction between the Western concept of divination and the African concept of divination. A typical example of the Western concept of divination sees divination as the endeavor to obtain information about things future or otherwise removed from ordinary perception by consulting informants other than human (Rose, 1975: 775). Middleton (1963: 196) defines divination as the attempt to discover events that do or will affect human beings for good or evil, but that are beyond their control and believed to have supernatural, mystical other than human cause. These definitions do not fit Emu conceptualization of divination, and associated practices. To the people of Emu, divination is not solely targeted at knowing the will of some far removed deity on human destiny, neither is all about learning the present or future. In Emu community, divination is used by the medicine man when dealing with clients. The goal then is to diagnose the clients' condition and obtain remedy.

4.7.1 Classification of Medicine and Ritual Practices in Emu

There are basically four broad categories of medicine and ritual practices in Emu. They are productive, therapeutic, protective and destructive medicines. These different medicines and their enumerated and described in the following sub-sections.

4.8 Productive Medicine

4.8.1 Ogwu Afia-Okeawuli: (Medicine for Trade)

As indicated already in the introduction to this work, formal trading is only a recent innovation in the Emu community. It emerged as the result of cultural interaction between Emu and her neighbors. As Emu people became involved with market economy, they exchanged their agricultural produce for money. Invariably the need to boost trade and make profit became important. In other to ensure sales and profit, *Ogwu Afia-Okeawuli* (medicine for trade) is used. The ingredients for the preparation of the *Ogwu Afia-Okeawuli* according to the informant, Chijioke Oshilim (1990) are as follows:

1. *Effifia alulunta* (translation withheld by oral source)
2. *Si Ejuani* (head of a snake)
3. *Nkpo ezegu* (white eagle feather)
4. *Ebulugo* (parrot feather)
5. *Efeluche* (sand from the entrance of the market)
6. *Ntu* (ashes from the hearth that have stayed overnight)
7. *Nchaoji* (black native soap)
8. *Ego ayaka ise* (five cowries)

These items are put in a mortar and then pounded to a point where the ingredients could be molded into a ball. During the pounding of the ingredients, the *dibie* blesses the ingredients with *Nzu* (local white chalk) and recites the following incantations;

> *Kene bu ogwu afia-okeawuli ife oso mmalu be ele bee onomie yuso legbane ifei, onye oso nomieni yabe-ele* (This is medicine for trade. Another trader's goods must not sell before yours when they sit around you. Only you would sell. If your goods are not all sold, other people having their goods near you would not sell).

This incantation is recited simultaneously as the above listed ingredients are pounded in a mortar. The processed items are molded into a ritual medicine soap with which the client bathes before going to the market. While bathing, the client is required to recite the same incantations that the *dibie* uttered while preparing the soap. This particular medicine is also attested among *Umu-Onicha* people. There is however, a preference for animal ingredients by the *Umo-onicha* people, rather than herbs which are used by the Emu people. The *Umu-Onicha* people in administering the ritual medicine make use of the parched ingredients in the form of powder that is rubbed on the face and at the same time reciting the incantation.

4.8.2 Ogwu Isorlu Ibe Mmalu: (Medicine for Love)

There are different types of medicine for love in Emu. There are those medicines whose ends are to help an intending husband secure the love and affection of a chosen partner. Likewise, there are those for single ladies to win the heart of a lover. There exist other forms of medicine to gain the love of a woman against her will and another for amorous men to copulate with women who will not be conscious of the act until the affair had been consummated. According to an informant the commonest of this type is *Ogwu isorlu ibe Mmalu*. It is prepared with the following ingredients

1. *Efifia odu-ngwele* (translation withheld by oral sources.)
2. *Anu-ngwele tukulu* (translation withheld by oral sources.)
3. *Efifia kepuni neebe igbe esuesu igbijele di* (leaves that have sprout where red ants cluster)
4. *Ife nde ewu gekoamu omubusa* (placenta of a goat)
5. *Efifia achachi igunu* (translation withheld by oral sources.)
6. *Efeluche* (parrot feather)
7. *Igoni* (small padlock)

To prepare the portion, all these items, except the padlock, are thrown together in a mortar. They are then pounded until they become fine like powder. During the pounding process, Nzu is sprinkled into it while reciting the following verse:

> *Si elnuodi si oyeye kim-nacho, Oyeye kim-nacho, ni ewem oyeye. Si efeluch ekwomali ni ikpo ebuba. Si oyeye m nacho yabe lu y'eka kpo efa oyeye ke.* (As it is now, it's a woman that I am looking for; it is a woman that I am looking for. I do not have a woman. It is true that the parrot feather is not difficult to find in the mist of other feathers. Let the woman I am looking for, come to me).

The thread that women use to plait hair is used to tie the ingredients to a padlock. With this ritual padlock in his pocket the man visits the woman of interest. When he sees her, he unlocks the padlock and says the following words to the woman:

> I like you, I want you to be my friend and my lover. I want to marry you. You must have no objection.

After uttering these words, the man locks the padlock thus lucking in her will. In the hours that follow, specifically shortly before dawn, the woman will become increasingly restless, and eventually overpowered with the thought of the man who had told those words to her. Besides herself, she will pack her belongings and move in with the man. This medicine, like the Yoruba *Amudo*, fills the woman with sensual and amorous emotions and will render her incapable of resisting sexual advances from the man whose single motive for placing the charming on her was to sleep with her even against her will. The workings of *Isorlu ibe Mmalu* and *Amudo* differ and yet they have certain similarities. For the Yoruba *Amudo*, the intended lover's name is called when preparing the medicine in order to turn her heart to the supplicant. While for the Emu people, it is required that the user see the intended lover and tells her his desires and then luck her will into the padlock. The woman will only be free of the spell when the padlock is unlocked.

4.8.3 *Ogwu Akonuche*: (Medicine for Memory)

Ogwu Akonuche is used to aid and enhance memory. In the olden days, it was the prerogative of the priests and medicine men to use *Ogwu akonuche* in their onerous task of preserving religious traditions, ritual incantation, and numerous medicine prescriptions. Nowadays, it is used to commit to memory traditional songs and folklore like the *Igele* and *Uponda*. Recently, it is used by students to study for their examinations. The student using *Ogwu akonuche* for examination purposes must also study. According to my oral source, Chijioke Oshilim (1990), the following ingredients are needed to make the medicine:

1. *Nguta*	(translation withheld by source)
2. *Onunuokpete esa*	(7 leaves of sugar cane)
3. *Epelete*	(mouse)
4. *Ntolo*	(a fish)
5. *Ofu ose oji*	(one alligator pepper)
6. *Ude aku*	(palm kernel oil)

These ingredients are gathered into a mortar, then pounded together until they turn into a pastry\liquid substance. The mixed substance is stored in a small bottle, *Akpi ntikili*, and is licked by the client on a daily basis. While being ingested, the client utters the following incantations:

> *Ife nmalifu amali, batanifu nishi. Yaba pushiwe ndende, ife mmalifuni, yaba pushi ni uche-m, Nodi, feli nu uche ndende.* (The thing that I have already learnt and understood; which has entered my head, must not leave my head at all, at all. What I have learnt, must never leave my brain. It must stay in my brain forever).

At the time of the preparation, the incantation is not recited. It is recited only when the client ingests the substance. An incision is also made to the forehead of the client into which the pastes is rubbed. Analogous medicine is found among the Yoruba of Nigeria, they call it, ogun *isoye*. *Akonuche* is believed to cure absentmindedness and poor memory. It is also suggested by the *dibie* that for examination purposes, the pen should be treated with the medicinal paste before using it to write any examination. However, unlike the *Ogun isoye*, the *akonuche* does not influence the examiner to be generous in marking the exam written with a pen laced with *akonuche* medicine. Its only purpose is to aid the memory of the user.

4.8.4 *Ogwu Mmili:* (Rain Medicine)

According to one of my subjects, Idonor Isakpa (1990), the Emu people have two types of rain medicine: *Ogwu ifemmili* (medicine to ward off rain), it is used to prevent rainfall during important ceremonies such as burial ceremonies, and *Ogwu idommili* (medicine to cause rainfall); this is used to cause rainfall. Rain medicine could be classified as productive medicine depending on the purpose for which the rain is solicited. *Ogwu idommili* is rarely practiced in the community since the town is situated near the rain forest region and thus records abundant rainfall throughout the year. Naturally, *Ogwu ifemmili* is the most widely used rain medicine in the community. Thus, the use of *Ogwu Idommili* can only be for destructive purposes and for that reason, it falls outside the scope the productive category.

For balance, *Ogwu ifemmili* can also be used for destructive purposes. For example, it is said that some time ago, a renowned *dibie* from a neighboring community was brought to prevent rainfall during the instalment of the new *Okpala Uku* (the oldest and the leader of the council of elders; the ruling body) of the community. The period coincided with the planting season when yam seedlings have just been planted. The *dibie* as expected, prepared a powerful medicine which he, unknown to the people, short with bow and arrow into a coconut tree. However, after the ceremonies were successfully completed the *dibie* left for his town and everybody expected normal rainfall. But there was no rainfall; after many weeks, the newly planted yam seedlings and other crops in the farm began to wither. And there was famine that year. Another diviner was called to explain the cause of the problem. The diviner told the community that the *dibie* had a grievance against them and had planned to punish them by shooting the medicine to the top of a coconut tree. Immediately, the medicine was removed from the treetop there was a heavy rainfall. Emu people believe that rain makers can spoil social occasions, burial ceremonies, and festivals out of jealously. In Emu, a *dibie* could possess the skills to make and ward off rain, but one rarely practices both. According to my oral source, Idonor Isakpa, the following ingredients are required to prepare the *Ogwu Idommili*:

1. *Ugba*	(small branch of oil beans tree)
2. *Anwiliwa*	(translation withheld by oral source)
3. *Iddo*	(colony of red ants)
4. *Ichite*	(grass)
5. *Uda*	(spice)
6. *Nchete*	(translation withheld by oral source)
7. *Epia*	(translation withheld by oral source)

The first items are tied together and hung atop a slow burning fire. The second set of items are tired together and hung atop the same slow burning fire. One piece of a three-lobed kola-nut is chewed in the mouth with some little quantity of local gin and intermittently spat at the tied items with the following words:

> *Mbubu bu nchete ndende awulu; Mmili swe nuzoeya; Anwu ku mchoni, achonim mmili.* (*Nchete* does not grow on wood at all. Let the rain fall in far distance; let the sky be cleared of the rain cloud. Let the sun shine continually. It is only sun I want, I do not want rain).

In the process of slowly heating the tied items, a lot of smoke is produced. This smoke is blown in the direction of the town upon which the *dibie* wants the rain to fall. As the smoke is blown, incantations are made; the kola-nut is chewed and mixed with gin in the mouth. This mixture is spit on the items hanging above the fire. The *dibie* must not drink water. He drinks only the local gin; a violation of this rule renders the medicine ineffective.

Ogwu ifemmili only stave off rainfall. The medicine only becomes ineffective if the *dibie* drinks water. In Umu–Onicha the *dibie* is forbidden from bathing during the period of the ritual. It is observed from the above rituals that, there exist ideas of sympathetic medicine. The smoke that rises steadily from the burning wood are blown gradually as it rises towards the direction where the rain is commanded to fall instead of the community. It is believed that as the smoke is blown away so also the heavy rain cloud or rainfall.

4.9 Therapeutic Medicine

Therapeutic medicines are preparations used in connection with diseases, sicknesses, and generally to steer away evil forces. The efficacy of this medicine was cited by my sources as the reason why modern medical services in the Emu are hardly used. The number of clients that the *dibie* receives relative to the number that visits hospital lends credence to this assertion. Lack of use of modern health facilities has ultimately lead to the closure of the dispensary in the community. Fundamental to the avoidance of modern health facilities is the belief that most diseases and sicknesses, apart from their physical manifestations, have spiritual causes, as such they require spiritual interventions in the form of therapeutic medicine. The range of this medicine is vast, it includes the following:

4.9.1 Ogwu Efo-Olinwa: (Medicine for Stomach Ache)

Based on the information obtained from our informer, Oliver Abanum (1990), the following ingredients are employed in the preparation of the medicine for stomach ache:

1. *Uda*	(spice)
2. *Nwata-tunime* esu	(translation withheld by oral source)
3. *Nzu*	(local white chalk)

The *nwata-tunime esu* is removed from its tree with a cutlass and not by hand. This and other ingredients are put together in a mortar and then pounded until they turns into liquid. The liquid medicine is put into a bottle and mixed with some local gin. For immediate result, the patient is drinks half a glass of the mixture at 5 a.m. and half a glass at any other time as the patient wishes. The patient recites the following;

> *Emo nau dine efo obulu olinwa niafu ogwu na, ku ogwu kpolu osansogbu dine efo tufu ku ogwu ke lu olu.* (This sickness that is in my belly, be it gonorrhea, be it poison; even bellyache, when I drink this medicine, let it remove all the problems. Let the medicine work).

It is believed that when this medicine is ingested early in the morning, and the incantations uttered, the illness is cured immediately. Usually, the medicine is prepared only once for a patient. Any other subsequent administration of the medicine will lack the ritual power, unless the patient ties two *ego ayaka* (cowries) to the neck of the bottle that contains the medicine. It is only then that the potency will be retained even with subsequent addition of local gin into the ritual medicine in the bottle (Abanum 1990). The patient for whom the medicine is prepared is required to pay certain amount of money as demanded by the local custom. This payment is called *panyilee ogwu,* "raising of the medicine".

4.9.2 *Ogwu Ibele Orenu-ku*: (Medicine against Veneral Disease)

This ritual medicine serves dual purposes. The first and most common purpose is its use in the cure of venereal diseases. Its' second use is to cure miscarriage. According to Oliver Abanum (1990), the ritual medicine, when administered correctly, will first make the womb of a woman retain the fetus and preserve it from being aborted and invariably, the baby is carried to term. The medicine also eases labor pains; the woman in labor drinks it intermittently. The following are the ingredients and prescription for this medicine:

1. *Ayamba*	(translation withheld by oral source)
2. *Mgbalagu* ekobo	(root of coconut tree)
3. *Uda*	(spice)
4. *Mgbalagu obo nkilishi*	(lime root)
5. *Nwata tunime nesu*	(translation withheld by oral source)
6. *Mgbalagu ububa*	(translation withheld by oral source)
7. *Migbalagu abasi oji*	(root of kola-nut tree)

The above listed items are collected together and washed thoroughly. They are then cut into tiny bits with a knife that is not used for domestic purposes. The chopped items are gathered into a bottle and mixed with some local gin. The *Ego ayaka* are then tied with a string to the neck of the bottle. The concoction is stored overnight. After then, the medicine is ready for use. This medicine can be ingested at any time. However, like most curative medicines that are orally ingested, according to my informant, this medicine must be drunk in the morning. It is believed that diseases or sicknesses are inactive in the mornings. *Ogwu ibele orenu-ku* according to Abanum differs from *Ogwu efo olinwa* in the sense that, the only function of the latter is to cure stomach ache while the former serves the dual function of curing venereal diseases and preventing miscarriages. In the usage of *ogwu ibele orenu-ku* one does not only depend on recited words for its efficacy but also on the *Ego-ayaka*, tied to the neck of the bottle. This is to keep the potency of the medicine over time so that it can always be used. For *Ogwu efo olinwa,* a string of cowries is tied to the neck of the bottle as part of the whole procedure for preparing the medicine. A negation of this process mars the efficacy of the ritual medicine.

The general principle guiding the selection of medicinal properties in the preparation of therapeutic medicines in Emu community is the idea that behind every physical ailments and diseases there exist spiritual agencies. Therefore the roots, barks of trees, leaves, and herbs that are used in the preparation of these ritual medicines are believed to contain spiritual forces that can be instigated to fight off those malevolent forces that are responsible for such ailments. Studies by pharmacists affirm the medicinal properties of the root, leaves, and barks used in native medicines (Oliver Abanum, 1990).

Lastly, there are some other ritual medicines unlike the ones described above, whose ends are not to cure a particular disease or sickness *per se*. These particular ritual medicines are best described as medicines to control natural forces or evil forces. These ritual medicines have formed part of the heritage of the people, they are used purposefully and are approved by the community; therefore they are productive in a sense. The following are two types of this medicine.

4.9.3 *Ogwu Mmo Ni Mmalu Afu Enya*: (Medicine to Keep a Dying Man Awake)

For this medicine, the following ingredients are required:

1. *Mba-alibuzoto*	(translation withheld by oral source)
2. *Mbaoketu*	(translation withheld by oral source)
3. *Ntu-egbe*	(gun power)
4. *Alida*	(translation withheld by oral source)
5. *Nzu* (local white chalk)	(Peter Nwabefa 1990).

The first three items are to be put together in a mortar and pounded. Then the leaf called *Alida* is added and pounded together with the other ingredients. Lastly *Nzu* is sprinkled on the pounded substance. The concoction is then mixed thoroughly and molded into a "medicine ball," it is then ready for administration to a dying patient. Getting to the dying person, the medicine ball, which is held with the left hand, is crushed in the palm of the right hand and mixed together with water. The mixture is rubbed sparingly on the body of the dying person. Emu people believe that when rubbed on the body of an ill person, it makes them invisible to the spirit world and vice versa. Consequently, the dying person will not hear nor heed the call of death. This belief is line with African conceptualization of death as evil that intermittently visits the physical world. According to my informant, the efficacy of this ritual medicine could be reduced if oil is brought close to the place where the medicine is prepared (Nwabefa, 1990).

4.9.4 Ogwu Ikpefu Onwu Mmalu: (Medicine to Postpone Death)

In order to postpone death, *Owa Ikpefu Onwu Mmalu* is prepared using the following ingredients:

1. *Eze Kpume Kpume*	(translation withheld by oral source)
2. *Egbedi isiewo*	(translation withheld by oral source)
3. *Olimietolo*	(translation withheld by oral source)
4. *Okishi*	(triangular metal)
5. *Ebe eto oji*	(three lobe kola nut)
6. *Use oji*	(alligator pepper)

The first three of the listed ingredients are gathered, then compress and tied together with a white cloth. One piece of kolanut with three lobes is chewed thoroughly with some alligator pepper. Then the chewed kola-nut is smeared into the tied ingredients and the following words are recited.

> Ogwu na, yaba iduwu? *Yabu iduwa flu uno? Obulusi iduwu susu esu.* (This ritual medicine are you alive? Are you at home? Now, if you are alive and at home, give me sign).

It is believed that after reciting these words, the ritual medicine will immediately respond by the shaking violently the hand of the medicine. This will occur each time the words are chanted. If the above affirmative signs are absent, then it is believed that the medicine is not potent. If the medicine has been proved effective, it is showered with praises for responding actively. The white cloth containing the ritual medicine is then tied to the *Okishi* (triangular metal) and hung on top or under the bed of the dying man. This ritual medicine would keep the dying man alive. Except the rope suspending the ritual medicine is severed and falls to the ground the sick remains alive wasting, and decaying but still breathing (Nwabefa, 2003).

There is the story told about a very wealthy man in Emu, who was very influential and sought the help of a famous *dibie* to keep him alive with *Owa Ikpefu Onwu Mmalu*. However, this man suffered a stroke and became paralyzed from the head to the feet. He remained in this condition for nineteen years gradually decaying on his bed, refusing to die. All efforts to help him join his ancestors failed, since nobody except himself knew how to end his terrible condition. Nonetheless, a *dibie* was able to discern the cause of his condition and where to locate the medicine. When the children saw the ritual medicine under his bed, they immediately cut the rope suspending the ritual medicine and the sick man stopped breathing (Nwabefa, 2003). It is also believed that a man, who has this medicine hung in the corner of his room, will not meet with sudden death via spiritual attacks from his foes.

4.9.5 Ogwu Enya Enu: (Medicine to Cure Mental Illness)

Emu people have "medicine" to cure madness. The ingredients for this preparation are:

1. *Eddo*	(translation withheld by oral source).
2. *Ncha-oji*	(local black soap).
3. *Efifia kepuni ni inyi mmalu*	(leaves got from grave).
4. *Eya kepuni no ofi*	(sand collected with closed eyes).
5. *Efifia ni isi omi*	(leaves from the mouth of the well).
6. *Mmiri inakpo*	(snail water).
7. *Nkplu ego osisor*	(old form of money).

In order to prepare, the listed items are pounded together in a mortar except for the last item on the list. These ingredients must be pounded with the snail water. When the ingredients are thoroughly mixed from pounded, then the last item *npkuiu ego osisor* is added and pounded again together until the constitution turns into a medicinal paste. For use, this paste is rubbed in the eyes of a mentally ill patient in the mornings and evenings while muttering the following incantations: "*Enya lua ani, enya lua ani*" (be calm and regain consciousness). This particular ritual medicine is used only on mental patients.

4.9.6 *Ogwu emo na liali ne esu mmalu* (Medicine for Undefined Sickness)

Ogwu emo na liali ne esu mmaiu is designed to cure all those sicknesses that have eluded other preparations by forcibly ejecting them as urine or excreta. This medicine has wide range of functions and is believed to be more potent than those designed for specific ends. This medicine probably owes to religious change. The inability and failure of *Ogwu efo olinwa* and *Emo Uku* to effectively cure stomach diseases led to the emergence of *Ogwu emo na liali ne esu mmalu*. According to my oral source, the following ingredients are required for the preparation of this ritual medicine

1. *Alibosa*	(Onion).
2. *Copra*	(Nut).
3. *Uda*	(Spice).
4. *Uzziza*	(Spice).
5. *Nzu*	(Local white chalk).
6. *Ngede ne eefie*	(translation withheld by oral source).

To obtain the medicine, the afore-listed ingredients are gathered in large quantities and mixed together by pounding. During the process, the following words are recited:

> *Si emo di mmalu ne efo, ko dini ugbazu, ebe obune olafu ogwu na ke emo ke. Be sogbu sie, si ya yufu. Emo keu ni nsi, yu fua ni mma miri* (This sickness, be it in the stomach; Be it at the back, wherever, let this person not suffer from the sickness anymore. This person must excrete the sickness out of his body. This person must excrete the sickness through urine).

The pounded ritual medicine is then poured into a bottle and topped with water. This is different from *ogwu efo olinwa* and *Emo-uku* that is mixed with locally brewed gin. It is believed that if the mixture is mixed with alcohol instead of water and administered to an ill person, the patient will collapse and die. A glass of the ritual medicine is administered to the sick in the morning before breakfast and in the evening. This medicine will forcefully drive out the sickness and they will be expelled either by excretion or as urine. It must be noted that *Ogwu emo na liali ne esu mmalu*, unlike *Ogwu efo olinwa* and *Emo-uku* cannot be prepared by a lay medicine man who has knowledge of the ingredients and formula. It is only the *dibie* that has the sole power to make it effective. Unlike the other therapeutic medicines, the knowledge and power required to make this medicine effective is transferred from a *dibie* to a private medicine man through blessing, in order to equip such a person to undertake the preparation. This transfer of knowledge occurs with the *dibie* scooping some sand and then placing it in the palm of the recipient. It is only then that the efficacy of the medicine can be guaranteed when practiced by the private medicine man (Abigide 1990).

4.9.7 *Ogwu Iwofu Ngbashi*: (Medicine to Remove Poison)

This particular ritual medicine is tailored to nullify any poisonous substance that a patient must have ingested into his\her body. Its therapeutical and soothing effects endear it to mediciner and patients alike. According to my oral source, (Nwabefa 1990), this ritual medicine is prepared with the following ingredients:

1. *Efifia Nkpula amu ekite*	(translation withheld by source)
2. *Efifia ichite*	(translation withheld by source)
3. *Egedi ishiewo*	(translation withheld by source)
4. *Oji ebe efo*	(three lobe kola nut)
5. *Ose oji*	(alligator pepper)
6. *Nkulu uda eto*	(three sticks of spice)

The listed items are collected in a mortar and pounded together to a liquid substance. This ritual medicine's substance is given to the patient to drink very early in the morning. When this is ingested, all the poison, including such objects like nail, animal teeth and claw are dislodged from the body.

4.10 Protective Medicine

The Emu people, like every other African peoples, fear the power of destructive medicine. They are very aware of how these destructive forces could be employed by unknown persons at the slightest provocation or assumed wrong, to wreak havoc in their homes, families and even to unborn children. Besides the fear of evil medicine, the people believe that natural forces could manifest their powers in order to harm them. Therefore, numerous protective medicines are used to ward off both sources of evil. One of these protective medicines is *Ogwu nkpashi.*

4.10.1 Ogwu nkpashi: (Protection from Destructive Medicine)

According to my informant, (Michael Okuguni 1990), this medicine protects the user from poison. *Ogwu nkpashi* is specifically designed to protect the user from the destructive medicine known as *Igba npi* (the sending of poisonous objects into the body through psychic means). However, in a wider sense, *Ogwu nkpashi* offers protection against poisoned drinks or foods. The medicine is inserted, and resides, in the body of the user. From there, it sends out warning signals whenever it detects poison. If for instance the wearer of this medicine comes in contact with poisoned food, the medicine will cause the plate containing the poisoned food to vibrate and then shatter. The same will happen if to a glass that contains poisoned drink. If the user is doubtful and tries to eat or drink the poisoned substance, the described events will continue to occur (Michael Okuguni, 1990). The ingredients required to make this medicine are:

1. *Mmua esa* (seven sun fly)
2. *Ndidei* (earth-worm)
3. *Ntioke* (translation withheld by oral source)
4. *Nkpula-amu ekite* (translation withheld by oral source)
5. *Agamebu* (translation withheld by oral source)

These items are collected in a mortar where they are pounded together. The pounding must occurs in an open space and the following incantations are uttered in the process:

> *Kene, obulusi ngbashi di ni mmayi; Kobu tili, ntie eka; ya goshim si ne ife dini nh kobu mmaya. Obulu si njeko ja bulu mmaya Ia, si iko ke ya gbakpofu.* (Listen medicine, listen, if there is poison in my drink or food; if I touch it, let it show me that it is present, as I try to eat or drink it, let the glass explode).

At the end of such an utterance the medicine is blessed with *Nzu.* A new razor blade is used to make an incision into the middle finger of the two hands of the client and the ritual medicine is rubbed into the incision. However, the efficacy of the medicine could be nullified when the user drinks palm wine. It is therefore, requested that the user abstains from drinking palm-wine.

4.10.2 *Aju Ogwu*: (Medicine against General Poison)

In order to prepare the medicine that protects from poison, the ingredients listed below are procured.

1. *Ekwa okuku ukwuani esa*	(seven eggs from a local fowl)
2. *Ekumaki*	(termites)
3. *Ogbenwaeku*	(young palm tree)

The young palm tree is pounded into a pulp; the termites and eggs are then mixed into it. The resulting substance is used in two ways: First, it may be dried and molded into a ritual medicine for external use only. To use, a bit of it is crushed and mixed with water. The resulting paste is then rubbed on the affected body parts (Abanum, 1990). Secondly, it may be prepared as a drink by dissolving the dried medicine in water. When a subject drinks it, the person becomes immune to poisons. According to my source, the potency of this ritual medicine could be diluted if a rat touches it or if it is touched with oil. The ritual medicine must not be taken to the farm or where crops are planted. It is believed that *aju ogwu* emits psychic forces that will cause plants and crops to wither away. Thus, it has destructive and preventive functions.

There is another type of *aju ogwu* that does not have the described destructive side effects when it is misused. This medicine specifically targets the parts of the body (such as sore or swollen limbs) that may have been attacked with poison. Similar to the first *aju ogwu,* it can be drunk or applied externally to a poisoned area of the body. The ingredients for this medicine include the following:

1. *Oke etu*	(translation withheld by oral source)
2. *Anyamgba*	(roots)
3. *Nzu*	(local white chalk)
4. *Uda*	(spice)
5. *Nnuike*	(potash (salt))

To prepare this medicine, the listed items are gathered into a mortar and pounded together. The resultant mixture is mixed with water that the user drinks in order to obtain its preventive power. The medicinal substance could be left to dry for storage. When its protection is required, portion of it is mixed with water to form a paste that is rubbed on the affected body part.

4.10.3 Ogwu Nkpokwa: (Antidote for Destructive Medicine)

Ogwu nkpokwa is one of the most widely used potions against attacks from destructive medicine. It is a mixture that protects the user from evil intentions of their enemies. These enemies may be sorcerers, witches, private and professional medicine men who, due to their knowledge, could conjure destructive medicine against a person. Thus, people seek *Ogwu nkpokwa* to ward off any spiritual attack directed towards them. The ingredients are:

1. *Anagba-enyawu nu ututu, enyawu ne cyashi*	(bark of Iroko tree)
2. *Ubili*	(bark of a tree)
3. *Ugba*	(bark of oil beam tree)
4. *Ogilishi-enyawu nu ututu, enyawu ne eyashi*	(bark of neoboldia tree)
5. *Isi npu*	(head of an animal)
6. *Isi abor*	(head of an animal)
7. *Okuku okpa*	(a cock\rooster)
8. *Ugbugbe*	(small cooking pot)
9. *Nzu*	(local white chalk)

These items are pounded together in a mortar until they turn into a pulp. During the pounding process, the mediciner recites the following incantations as he blesses the preparation with *Nzu* (Abanum, 1990).

> *Nkpokwa! we kpo anagba; Anagba ne shi osa ife we no nelo ni-rn njo; Ya kpokala tufu gbu me egbu, onye kunisi ojeke gbu me egbe, o telu- ukom ndende. Onu kuni njo ya neku nma* (Nkpokwa! When you call the Iroko tree, it must answer you. It does not reject a call. All the bad things that people conceive against me must be gathered together and thrown away. Whoever says he will kill me would never get to me, at all, at all. The lips that speaks ill, will also speak good.).

The now pounded ingredients are transferred to *ughugbe* (a small cooking pot). The heads of *npu* and *abor* (animals) are placed on top of the ingredients in the pot. Thereafter, the rooster is slaughtered and the *nkpokwa* medicine in the *ugbugbe* is doused with the blood of the slaughtered rooster and left to ferment overnight. At dawn, as the cock crows, incision is made on the forehead of the user and the ritual medicine is rubbed into the incision. *Ogwu nkpokwa*, like the Yoruba's *Madarikon*, is believed to shield an individual from destructive medicine directed against the user. Also, like *madarikon*, it is believed that *Ogwu nkpokwa* not only prevents attacks from witches and workers of evil medicine, it can return the evil medicine to the sender. However, *Ogwu nkpokwa* differs from the Yoruba *madarikon* that in addition to shielding the user from evil, it renders the user invisible to evil medicines and attacks. *Ogwu nkpokwa* does none of these. In Ghana, there is a similar ritual medicine that is used to protect the user from evil medicine (Neal 1985). According to Neal, before he was attacked by evil medicine in the form of a "bad snake", he had sought the protection of a medicine, likened to *Ogwu nkpokwa*. He reported two remarkable experiences. "The sudden stopping of the "bad snake", and the splitting of a perfectly healthy tree into two halves. Each half then stood a foot or so apart from the spots where *Malam Alargi* had buried his protective medicines" (1958: 15). *Ogwu nkpokwa* is designed to operate similar to Neal's experience. The difference between the two forms of protective medicines is that the former is buried around the house to protect the user from evil medicine, while *Ogwu nkpokwa* is rubbed into an incision on the forehead of the user.

4.10.4 *Ogwu Ashima*: (Medicine that grants Premonition)

It is a common practice among the *Emu* people to employ "intuitive signs" in their daily decision making processes. These signs may be positive or negative. They help the people to take decisions such as; whether or not to travel; whether or not to go to the farm; and whether or not to engage in a particular business venture. According to the people, when such signs are ignored, the consequences are always serious. Thus, it is common to hear Emu person say that the palm of his\her is itching. To them, this is a sign that signifies that some money might soon come his\her way. They take a twitch in the left hand as a warning that, their contemplated plan might come to naught if embarked upon. However, in cases where there is a preponderance of such signs, the *dibie* is consulted. According to my informant, Onyenajua (1990), the recipe for *Ogwu ashima* is as follows:

1. *Onunuokpele esa* (7 leaves plucked at the road side)
2. *Againebu* (translation withheld by informant)
3. *Ofu ose oji* (alligator pepper)
4. *Eju agama* (pubic hair of a woman)

These items are gathered together in a mortar and pounded into a smooth powder. During the pounding process the following incantations are recited:

> *Ibe nobune odine; odine nume ute ki idie ani; Odini ni ime etiti imenge de; Odini hu ututu, si ashima beye. Si eka elife bulu ko-oma, eka ekpe bulu ko-ojo Njeko ogoshim. Ogwa si ku-mbe ye, Ijewe. Ome ko-ojo, ijekom Ome ko oma ejem ebe nyeko.* (Wherever I may be, be it in the middle of the night when I am sleeping or be it in the morning time, let *ashima* give me a sign. Let the right hand be a good sign and the left hand be a bad sign. Wherever I am going let it show me a sign. If it tells me not to go I will not go. If it gives me a good sign I will go to where I am supposed to go. Let ashima give me a sign.).

The resulting medicinal powder is divided into two equal sides. The *ufie* (local dye) is mixed into the half that is to the right side of the mediciner and *ntu* (gun powder) is mixed into the potion on the left. These are then mixed together. With a razor blade incisions are made to the base of the left and right arms. The ritual powder is rubbed into the incisions. Now the user is fortified and will always be informed through jerking, scratching or shaking of the arm or palms about the appropriateness or not of an intension. In this culture, omens to the left hand are bad omens, and those to the right, are good.

Ogwu ashima works for all users, it does not discriminate based on the purpose for which it is used, whether it is for armed robbery or not. Nonetheless, there are conditions that will render *Ogwu ashima* inaccurate. Rain or wet conditions reduces the potency of *Ogwu ashima*. Wet conditions are said to encourage the power inherent in the medicine to slumber. To remedy this limitation, it is recommended for users who live or work under such wet or rain conditions, to eat bitter kolanut and drink some local gin while reciting the incantations at least once a day. Doing this will keep 'awake' the *Ogwu ashima*.

4.10.5 Ogwu Njo Puazo: (Medicine to Avert Evil Forces)

Ogwu njo puazo works for the user to avert all evils including those caused by natural forces. Unlike the *Ogwu nkpokwa* and the Yoruba *madarikon* that prevents attack from evil medicines, *Ogwu njo puazu* prevent the user from encountering physical, natural or spiritual evils. As the name implies, all troubles must occur in the absence of the user. If evil must occur it will be before the arrival or after the departure of the user. According to my informant, Peter Nwabefa (1990), the following ingredients are needed for the preparation of this ritual medicine:

1. *Ekwukwo olimajini ughazu puezuku esa*	(seven leaves the back of which faced the road)
2. *Akpashi ke dm1 ani uno esa*	(seven broomsticks picked from the floor of the house)
3. *Ichite*	(grass)
4. *Ekwukwo*	(leaves)
5. *Ekwukwo efeluche*	(leaves)
6. *Nkpulu esu*	(bead)
7. *Npi ngbada*	(horn of an antelope)

The first four items are gathered into a mortar and pounded into a paste using only local gin as mixture. To this preparation, the remaining items are added and then pounded together again. After this, a razor blade is used to cut incision to the mouth and the forehead of the client. Then the medicinal substance is rubbed into these cuts (Nwabefa 1990). Unlike the other protective medicine, *Ogwu njo puazu* does not require any incantation. The efficacy of this medicine does not hinge on the power of the spoken word. It is believed that the medicinal ingredients when properly and normatively combined are inherently powerful to achieve its end for the user. *Ogwu njo puazu* is also different from the other protective medicine, in the sense that its power is not eroded or diminished by certain restrictions or taboos. In *Ogwu njo puazu*, we are able to see ideas of imitative medicine. Interestingly, among the ingredients is the 'broom' that the people use to sweep inside (not outside) their house. The under-lying idea is that, as the broom sweeps away dirt, so also the medicine will sweep away all evils that might befall the user. The broom thus symbolizes the cleaning away of evils. The *npi ngbada* (horn of an antelope) is another instance of imitative medicine. The antelope is recognized in the community as an animal that is quick to run away from trouble. Therefore, it is believed that the user will always be ahead of trouble or evil.

The experience of Chief Okponku, a businessman who holds a traditional title in the community illustrates the working of this medicine. In 1989, he had wanted to embark on his routine business trip to Onitsha to purchase building materials for his store in Emu. But on the day of his trip, he changed the time of his departure from his usual 9 a.m. to noon. He also decided to use public transport instead of his van. On returning from his trip, he met members of his household in a mourning mood and was informed that his elder brother who had taken the van out that day and at the time was murdered by armed robbers. The robbers made away with his money and the van: However, when one member of the robbery gang was apprehended he confessed that they had intended to rob and kill Chief *Okponku* and not the unfortunate man that became their victim, Later, when this writer asked the Chief if he had a fore-knowledge of the incident, shaking his head he responded, how could he had known and not warn everyone not to use the van. He however confirmed that he had *Ogwu njo puazo* cut into his body by a powerful *dibie*, and that is why he went at noon instead of his usual 9 a.m. He confessed later, that the sad incidence was not the first misfortune he had escaped (Okponku, 1990).

4.10.6 Ogwu Mma: Preotective Medicine against Cutlass and Knife attacks (1)

Apart from the medicine that protects the user from untold happening and evil or mystical attacks, there are other forms of protective medicine that are believed to safeguard the user from weapons such as cutlass, knife, and gun. These types of medicine that make the user invulnerable to sharp objects and gunshot had been in use since the founding of the community. During the days of migration Emu engaged in wars with neighbors and enemies alike. In these wars, every able bodied men were expected to participate in defending the community or in expanding its' frontiers. The people naturally sought means of protection against their enemies' weapons. Thus, *Ogwu mma* (cutlass medicine) and later *Ogwu egbe* (gunshot medicine) were developed. The ingredients for this protective medicine are:

1. *Ekpa esu-esu*	(nest of soldier ants)
2. *Okpa*	(cock)
3. *Nkpili-ite*	(local pot)
4. *Ekpilikpa akambor*	(shell of a porcupine)
5. *lkpokili-inakpo*	(empty shell of snail)
6. *Esu akpulosa*	(shell of a tortoise)

According to my informant, when collecting the nest of the soldier ants, "you go along with the cock at sun rise and later in the evening, at sunset. Cut the stem of the leave housing the ants into a paper bag. Then make a fire with a tripod stand upon which the local pot is mounted. In this pot you put in the ants, shell of a porcupine, shell of a snail and tortoise. Then you cut the leg of the cock and let the blood drip into the pot. These ingredients are allowed to heat and get burnt in the pot". The residue becomes the ritual medicine that is used on the clients. Some of the burnt medicinal ingredients are eaten, while the rest is rubbed on the chest and back of the user. A ring could also be added to the medicinal substance and heated together. This ring is then worn as charm to protect the user from cutlass and knife cuts. However, a person in possession of this type of medicine is not allowed to eat *mmu egwa* (small beans) or squat to cook. The user must always keep the head of his cutlass in an upright position. Even when somebody else's cutlass is seen heads' down, the user of *Ogwu mma* must pick the cutlass up, wave it around his head three times, and return it heads' up. A negation of this will reduce the efficacy of the medicine. This medicine needs no incantation. It is in of itself potent enough as long as its restrictions and taboos are kept. The idea of imitative medicine is also evident in the use of hard shells of animals in these prescriptions. Just as the shell protects the animal inside it, so will the user of *Ogwu mma* be made hardened against sharp objects and protected from them.

4.10.6b Ogwu Mma: Protective Medicine against Cutlass and Knife attacks (2)

The ingredients for this second type of medicine are:

1. *Mgbalagu Inene*	(root)
2. *Otogbu lugbu*	(leaves)
3. *Ekwa okukwu uno*	(egg from local fowl)

4. *Ulu une* (rotten pulp of plantain stem)
5. *Njanja* (leaves)
6. *Udor* (local rope)
7. *Egba* (large arm metal ring)
8. *Nwa ugbu'gbe* (small local pot)
9. *Ofigbo* (palm oil)

The items are gathered together in a mortar. Only a girl below the age of ten is allowed to pound the ingredients. During the pounding the *dibie* blesses the ingredients with *nzu* saying but not reciting that, "The person (name of client) for whom the medicine is being prepared must not be hurt by cutlass or knife". These words do not have any power on their own. Hence the absence of these words does not negate or improve the efficacy of the medicine. Although, it is believed that medicine knows its owner, it is assumed that the words spoken are a kind of identification of the owner with the medicine, since the words are said while blessing of the ingredients with *nzu*.

The pounded ingredients are scooped into the small pot which also contains the metal arm ring. This is left to soak overnight. The following morning the metal arm ring will be ready for use. This metal arm ring is to be kept at all times in the pot containing the medicinal ingredients and from there taken for use when necessary. The ring is worn on the left arm. It is believed that a person having this medicine can never be hurt by cutlass or knife in the event of war or if attacked with sharp objects. Unlike the first *Ogwu mma,* where a machete or knife is treated with medicine that is rubbed into an incision, it is believed that the user of this *Ogwu mma* will not be harmed by such cutlasses or knives laced with medicine. Lastly, the efficacy of this second type of *Ogwu mma* will be nullified if the user has sexual intercourse while wearing the medicinal metal ring.

4.10.7 Ogwu Mma Nbubu: Medicine against Cutlass Medicine

The ingredients for this medicine include the following:

1. *Onunu okpete esa* (seven leaves)
2. *Ekwukwo ugba* (leaves of oil bean tree)
3. *Ekwa okuku esa* (seven local fowl eggs)
4. *Ofu ogbe ose oji* (one alligator pepper)
5. *Ofu nkpulu uda* (a stick of spice)

These items are gathered into a mortar where they are pounded together. During the pounding, the mixture of the ingredients is blessed with *nzu* with the following words, "The cutlass that is laced with anti-cutlass medicine, *Ogwu mma nbubu*, must surely cut anybody that has the cutlass medicine". Then the pounded medicinal mixture is cut into the body of the user via incision. The cutlass that the user intends to use in an attack or war is also laced with the medicine. This cutlass must not be used for farm work or domestic duties or by any other person. It must be used by the owner into whose body the incision was made and only for war against enemies that are assumed to have supernatural immunity from cutlass and knife cuts. This medicine is socially approved by the community and therefore does not fit into the category of destructive medicine. *Ogwu mma nbubu* provides protection to the community and against destructive to the enemy. Since this medicine is made against external aggressors, it is believed that if it used against an indigene or members of the Emu community, it will become impotent and not successful.

Under protective medicine against cutlass cuts, are numerous other types of medicine that are outside our scope of this work. For example, medicinal protection for a single day would entail chewing and swallowing of *okpete* leaves with seven seed of alligator pepper, or seven leaves of *esisa*, seven pieces of broom sticks, and seven seeds of alligator pepper or seven leaves of *ngba-borchi* and seven seeds of alligator pepper. It is believed that when any of the recipes above is followed, the user would be protected from cutlass and knife cut for one day. Nonetheless, the user's cutlass or knife must not be seized and used against them by the enemy as the day's medicine will not offer protection against own instrument.

4.10.8 Ogwu Egbe Ufie: Medicine against Wounds Sustained from Gunshot

To prepare potions that protects against gun shot, the following ingredients are needed.

1. *Ofu efele* (one plate)
2. *Ofu okpe* (one cock)
3. *Obianofu* (leaves)

4.	*Odu oghene*	(coco-yam tuber)
5.	*Ite*	(hollow drinking pot)
6.	*Egba*	(metal arm ring)
7.	*Udeaku*	(oil from fried kernel)
8.	*Ofu ngbor*	(one cartridge)
9.	*Okpete*	(translation withheld by informant)
10.	*Omu egbe ndeaka*	(ancient form of bullet)

The medicine is obtained by placing *udu oghene, obianofu,* and the content of the cartridge into the pot. The seven *okpete* leaves, which must be uprooted in one motion from the ground, are added. The *udeaku* is mixed with water in a plate. Then one of the legs of the rooster is cut and its blood is let to drip into the mixture, and then the metal arm-ring is inserted into the pot. A razor blade is used to cut two incisions to each of the breasts, make two incisions to each side of the waist. The content of the plate is then sprinkled on the incisions and all parts of the body. This pot, with its contents, which must be on a tripod stand, is kept in a corner of the bedroom. The pot must be left without a lid (uncovered) at all times and no water must get into the pot (Chukwukuni, 1990).

When going to war, the metal arm-ring is retrieved from the pot. The body of the person going to war is rubbed with some of the medicinal ingredients from the pot. A person wearing these metal rings will become invulnerable to gunshots. The bullet will be shot at the user with accompanying sound but the bullet will be deflected from the user *wu egbe ufie.*[1]

Another type of medicine that offers protection against gunshot is *Elieli gba nwata oseleaka.* According to my oral source, Chukwukuni (1990)

1 I witnessed a demonstration of this medicine during the *Igbu* festival where protective medicine against cutlass and gunshots are usually tested among the warlords of the community. Two pots were brought out one containing the medicine and the other not. Guns were fired at both randomly, the one pot without the charm was shattered but not the one containing the medicinal ingredients. One of the participants brought out of the pot the metal arm ring and pinned it to a plantain stem. Guns were fired at the plaintain stem repeatedly wihout effect.

the following ingredients are employed for the preparation of this kind of ritual medicine;

1. *Mgbo*	(cartridge)
2. *Afamla*	(translation withheld by informant)
3. *Atapia*	(translation withheld by informant)
4. *Onunu oka-Efifia kepuni mmiii esa*	(7 leaves that brings out water)
5. *Ulankita*	(translation withheld by informant)
6. *Ekwukwo ugba*	(leaves of oil bean tree)
7. *Ekwukwo awuinwa*	(translation withheld by informant)
8. *Ekwukwo kponkpu*	(translation withheld by informant)

To prepare this medicine, all the afore-listed items are gathered together in a mortar and pounded. The resulting mixture is allowed to dry and is then set ablaze. As the dried pounded medicinal ingredients are burning, they are blessed with *nzu* and with the following words:

> *Si we gba ye egbe si ngbo, ba beyenesu, si osa ngbo beluye esu, belu ebeidi. Si we bule egbe tua, onyeu da na ani.* (When a gun is shot at you, let the bullet not enter the body. Let none of the bullets reach where you are. When a gun is shot at you, let it lift up your assailant in the air and throw him to the ground).

The medicine loses its efficacy if a menstruating woman touches it or comes near where it is been prepared. When it is ready, a razor blade is used to cut seven incisions into the chest of the user and four to the back. The burnt medicinal ingredients are rubbed into the cuts (Chukwukuni, 1990).

The *Ogwu egbeufie, Ogwu elieli gba nwata* oseleaka was tested by the *dibie* himself during the recent inter-village war between *Ogume* and Emu community. During the fight, according to him, he played a prominent role by leading the group of warriors that were firing guns. At the front-line where he was giving orders to his group, gunshots were fired continually at him, none of which touched him. Unfortunately, some members of his ranks, behind him who were not protected with this medicine died (Chukwukuni, 1990). The difference between *Ogwu egbeufie* and *Ogwu elieli gba nwata* is that the former stops the bullet from reaching the one wearing the protective medicine. The latter causes the attacker to lose aim and balance. Sometimes, it throws the attacker high up into the air and then dashes him to the ground.

Emphasis is not placed on the spoken words during the preparation of *Ogwu egbe*. This is because the forces residing in the ingredients are powerful enough to make the user immune to gunshots. However, the user is expected to announce his goals to the medicine in the pot before using it. Different from this is *Ogwu elieli gba nwata oseleaka* that lays great emphasis on the power of the spoken word in addition to the power that is inherent in the medicinal ingredients. Unlike the *Ogwu egbe ufie*, one does not need to arouse the medicine by announcing his intention for its use. It is believed that *Ogwu egbe ufie* is always awake and alert at all times (Chukwukuni, 1990).

4.11 Destructive Medicine

Destructive medicines are those types of medicine that are injurious towards humans, properties, and the society in general. This type of medicine is commonly described as evil or bad medicine because it could be used to disrupt the harmony of individuals, homes, and business. Unlike other varieties already identified, Emu people think that destructive medicine is seldom used. Professional and lay-medicine men could use this medicine to wreak havoc on people who had (unknowingly) offended them. It is feared that people with unstable and bad character could employ medicine men or themselves, to seek redress through destructive medicine either on perceived wrongs or out of spite or jealousy. Thus, in order not to be taken unawares, most of the people seek protection from various type of this medicine. However, knowledge of the recipes of destructive medicine is not easy to come by, since most medicine men claim ignorance of such medicine or sometimes are outright hostile. According to these medicine makers no serious minded person who has no evil intention towards another person will spend their time seeking the knowledge of this medicine. Giving this seeming rebuff from the practitioner, it is difficult to obtain information on destructive medicines beyond those few commonly spoken about in the community.

4.11.1 *Ogwu Igba Nkpa*: (Poison)

Literarily, this medicine translates to "shooting poison". This medicine is usually employed in a fit of anger and with the intention to kill. *Ogwu Igba*

Nkpa acts instantly. According our oral source, Ifeaka Odinama (1990), the following ingredients are need in order to prepare the medicine:

1.	*Alili-nwusunini*	(Dead millipede)
2.	*Ntuku*	(Toad)
3.	*Ogumagada*	(Chameleon)
4.	Bottle *ntikpo*	(Broken pieces of bottle)
5.	*Ntutu*	(needle)
6.	*Obulogu*	(corrosive leaf)
7.	*Ekwukwo ogbome*	(translation withheld by oral source)
8.	*Ose oji*	(Alligator pepper)
9.	*Ude aku*	(Palm kernel oil)
10.	*Nkporuka*	(ring)

To obtain the medicine, all the listed items except for the ring and oil from kernel are gathered into a mortar, where they are pounded together. The resulting mixture in the put into a container to which are added the oil and the ring. These are then cooked on fire until all its liquid content are evaporated. With a razor blade incision is made into the middle finger of the user. The dried content is then rubbed into the incision. When the cut is healed, the ring is worn on the same finger to which incision was made. To use, the finger with the ring is flickered thrice at the direction of an adversary; with this the poisonous ingredients are shot into the body of the adversary where it begins to destroy its victim. *Ogwu lgba-nkpa* is dangerous and if not immediately detected and nullified, it will lead to death (Ifeaka Odinama, 1990).

4.11.2 *Ogwu Eti Ada*: (Hit and make a person fall to the ground)

This type of medicine is widely used among the youths and people who might have reason to engage in physical fights. The medicine helps the user to subdue an opponent in a fight. As the name indicates, when the victim is hit by the user, the victim will fall to the ground, and will be begin to convulse uncontrollably, scrapping the ground with his mouth. It is believed that if the victim is not rescued immediately by the assailant, the victim will die. The recipe for this medicine is as follows:

1. *Akuebenishi*	(translation withheld by informant)
2. *Enwupuku*	(giant flies)

3. *Elieli* (large black ants)
4. *Ite-tikponi* (broken pot)
5. *Egedi ishiewo* (translation withheld by informant)
6. *Agamebu* (translation withheld by informant)
7. *Mboagu* (translation withheld by informant)
8. *Nkponeakaabuo* (two rings)

To make this medicine, all the listed items are cooked together in a pot until they are burnt. With a razor blade seven incision marks are made into the wrist of the client and the burnt ingredient is rubbed into it. The ring is then worn on the third finger of the hand that has been incised. The hand with the ring must at all times be kept away from oil. Contact with oil makes the medicine lose its potency. It is, however, believed that the user of *eti-ada* must be the aggressor, he\she must only use it for self-defense. As long as it is in response, the use of this medicine is justified. A victim of this medicine can only be rescued either by the assailant or by a *dibie*. The antidote consists in some herbal bath. Generally, the community frowns at people who use this medicine even in the face of provocation. Usually, people caught using this type of medicine are heavily fined.

4.11.3 *Ogwu Ibo Mmalu Onti*: (Medicine to Cause Madness)

With this medicine, a person could be commanded to become crazy. The use of this medicine in the Emu community has been practically discontinued. In the past, it was employed only in extreme circumstances in order to severely punish an individual. The following are the ingredients of this medicine.

1. *Mgbalagu okesusu* (translation withheld by informant)
2. *Mgbalagu ose* (one seed of pepper)
3. *Mgbalagu otulu* (translation withheld by informant)
4. *Ofu nkpulu esu* (one centipede)
5. *Ekwa ododo* (piece of red cloth)
6. *Ofu egoayaka* (one cowry)
7. *Akwebinishi* (translation withheld by informant)

To obtain this medicine, items 1–3 are pounded separately. To this are added the rest of the ingredients and they are pounded thoroughly. To use, the client scoops some of the concoction into the mouth before sunrise, he\ she chews it while standing. Then pointing a finger at the early morning sun the user recited the following words:

> *Ifekene njekojeme oyene, obulusi ifekeni omeni tuluma atulu, si nchoni ki ela kua, ela na kua.* (This thing that I want to do to this person is because the wrong he did me (mention the wrong) really hurt me. So, I want him to run mad. Madness should overcome him. Madness must overcome him.).

The user spits out all the medicinal ingredients at once towards the morning sun. The same action is repeated the next two days consecutively at the same time. The person that the evil curse is directed at will become insane. His condition will worsen with each rising sun until he loses his senses completely (Nwabefa, 1990).

The Emu people believe, just like the Yoruba people, that the medicine of curse (*Ibo mmalu onu*) is the most common cause of mental disorder. Ibo *mmalu onu* can neither be used to bless people nor help a woman in labour to make delivery easy. It is regarded as an anti-social medicine. *Ibo mmalu onu* cannot be used without a prior knowledge of the victim's name. It also resembles the Yoruba *Isasi* medicine which is used to cause some confusion in a victim's life. The preparation of *Ibo mmalu onu* involves incantation, and the mentioning of the name of the victim as well as the affliction that is desired. The most important aspect of this medicine is the incantation, this has to be uttered correctly at the specified time of the day, facing the right direction and mentioning the victim by name.

4.11.4 *Ogwu Akpanya-ga* (Medicine to create confusion)

Emu's destructive medicine includes *Akpanya-ga,* that is, to scatter, that is to create confusion and disharmony. It operates on contact with the premises or surroundings of the intended victim. It could also have the same destructive effect on buildings, machinery or a place. To activate this medicine, it has to be thrown at or brought into contact with anything that connects to the intended victim. As soon as this happens, confusion will begin to reign in the life of the victim. Not until the medicine is discovered and removed will peace return to the premises or life of the victim. Below is the recipe for *Akpanya-ga,* as described by my informant:

The ingredients are:

1. *Nku otulu lefuni* (Rotten wood)
2. *Uda nkpulu esa* (Seven sticks of spice)
3. *Akwebinishi* (Bark and leaves that fell face up)
4. *Egbono* (Fruits picked at the rising and setting of the sun)

These items are gathered into a mortar where they are pounded and mixed together. During the pounding, *nzu* is sprinkled on it and the following incantation is recited:

> *Akpanya-ga! Siifekene inememe, si ntieye nunno mmalu, si unoke niniwu, si ntie ni ogo mmalu, ogo ke kpeye kolo. Si osa iji dino ogo kewu dufu okwu. Si Osa mmalaka dino ogokewu kpeye fu. Si we ba fu efeli, Akpanya-ga!* (This ingredient that I have prepared, when put in X's house, let there be confusion, if put in X's farm, let the farm be destroyed, that all the yams in the farm should get burnt; let all the cassava in the farm be destroyed, let X not see food to eat).

The resulting ingredients are tied together with a black rag and deposited in the victims' house or yard. If thrown into a farm, the crops in the farm will gradually wither or catch fire mysteriously, or sometimes they will get trampled by animals.

4.12 Medicine with dual functions

Lastly, in looking at the different types and categories of medicine there are those types that have dual functions. They could be put to good, positive or to bad, negative uses.

4.12.1 *Ogwu Iwa Ugboko*: Medicine of Command in the Forest

Below is the ingredients needed for the preparation of this kind of ritual medicine:

1. *Efifia ebekele ekwukwo esa* (Translation withheld by informant)
2. *Mgbalagu kedire enu* (root)
3. *Uyi oku* (ashes)
4. *Ntu egbe* (gun powder)
5. *Ekwukwo ododo* (red colored leaves)

The listed ingredients, except the last one, are gathered in a mortar and pounded together. While pounding, saliva is spit into the mortar containing the ingredient. The following words are to be recited while the pounding is going on:

> *Ifenkuni neu, ya me. Kene-ne yekeku bu ije ugboko. Nfu onyeke ibei flu ugboko, ngwa s (hei!) yemu mmai, oyeme. (hei!) yemu egbei, oyeme. Igwa si yabulosor gbabusa nu ugboko, obuloso gbabusa flu ugbokonu.* (Let whatever I say from my mouth happen. Whenever I see a fellow man in the forest and I say hei! Give me your cutlass. He will give it to me. Hei! give me your gun. He gives it to me. When I command him to run mad into the bush, he obeys. When I command him to run out of the bush, he will obey.).

When thoroughly mixed, the pounded medicinal ingredients are collected into *ekwukwo ododo* leaves and tied up and then sewn into a leather pouch that is worn like a necklace around the neck. When invoked, the medicine operates by causing a biting sensation to the navel and stomach of the user as a sign of an impending danger. The user thus has ample time to recite the incantation before an unfavourable encounter.

4.12.2 *Ogwu Odor*: (Medicine to Recall Someone)

Another type of medicine in this same category is *Ogwu udor*, it is used to recall someone who is abroad. Unlike the Yoruba *Ayogo* that is used to send a person out of town, this medicine is used in *Emu* to recall someone to Emu. The following is a recipe for making *Ogwu udor*:

1. *Ekwukwo nfud esa*	(translation withheld by informant)
2. *Ekwukwo ishi uku esa*	(translation withheld by informant)
3. *Efifia ose ani*	(translation withheld by informant)
4. *Ufie*	(dye)
5. *lIe okpa*	(cock's tongue)
6. *Ichite ke dine isuku*	(grass on the road side)
7. *Egbugba anagba*	(bark of the iroko tree)

All these items are collected together in a mortar and then pounded. *Nzu* is sprinkled on the mixture and the following words are recited:

> *Ebene obune oyekene dine (*name of the person*); Kene oju eluno, ife kene bu ifu-uya. Si nchoni kolu mm. Nodi lunno kolu, yabu efaya epusu. Si nchoni lolu uno. Si nyene ubochi eto oji lunno.* (Wherever this person (name of person) is, for

having not come back in a long time, we consider it a punishment on the family, a shame, a bad thing. I want him to come back home. If he does not come back, may his name be lost. I want him back home. He is given three days to come home).

The pounded medicinal ingredients are tied to the top of a bamboo pole and pinned to the ground, facing the east. As the morning sun appears, the user touches the ritual medicine, longing for the person who was summoned. It is believed that the instant the user touches the medicine, the person to whom it is directed will know that s\he is wanted back home urgently. Each day that action is repeated, the victim will become restless and greatly troubled, so much so that s\he must return home. "If he does not go home, he will not experience peace" (Nwabefa 1990). The efficacy of this medicine is never doubted by the Emu people. There was this incident, according to my informant, of his elder brother, who had refused to return home for about twenty eight years. Since his elder brother was needed for their late father's burial, my informant had no choice than to resort to this particular medicine to bring back the recalcitrant brother. Thus he followed scrupulously the prescription of this medicine and to his amusement, the elder brother returned home on the third day. On questioning, the elder brother confirmed that he was greatly troubled, but had no particular reason for coming home (Nwabefa, 1990).

There is another type of this kind of medicine, which is used in pinning down erring or wandering family member. This medicines involves mixing a medicinal herb called *kpanisheku-kpani-ani uno* into food. It is believed that whoever eats the food will lose every desire and interest to leave the community. These two types of medicine fall under the four main categories of medicine; productive, therapeutic, protective and destructive. How a medicine is classified depends on its use. As the brother of my informant argued, it is destructive to recall a man, against his will from his family and prosperous business abroad, only for him to come home and practice subsistence farming along with his kinsmen.

It is not a rule that all the ritual practices of the Emu people must solely depend on the medicinal ingredients in order to be effective. What is true from these studies thus far is that, some prescription like *Ogwu mma,* are equally effective without any formal incantation. On the other hand, most of the medicinal ingredients have some form of words that are not fixed nor necessarily spoken over the prescription in a form of a conversation.

For such, the medicine man can modify these words at his discretion. It has also been observed that, medicine as believed and practiced among the Emu people, is not just a set of mathematical formula which must achieve its results. Ritual rules and laws have a supernatural and mystical inference that binds the user. A violation of these rules or taboos will not only bring about a reduction in the potency of the medicine, but may have grievious consequences for the medicine man.

Chapter Five: Ritual Symbolism in Emu Ritual Practices

5.1 The Medicine Man

The most commonly and widely used Emu word to describe a traditional medicine practitioner is *dibie*. This is closely related to the Igbo usage. Among Igbo people, medicine is called *ogwu* and the medicine man is *dibia*. The word "*dibie*" equally stands for 'doctor' (qualified), "necromancer, and magician" (Basden 1938: 54). This understanding differs from the erroneous application of terms like "witch doctor" and "fetish doctor" by Europan-American writers to African medicine man (Mbiti 1969: 166). As suggested by lkenga-Metuh (1987: 221). If the word "fetish" means a bundle of some material objects believed to be capable of generating some mystical powers, then it is true that some medicines are 'fetish'. However, most African medicines are "not fetish at all."

The medicine man has been defined in various ways. Mostly according to his function and position in this society. The medicine man is a kind of scientist, in that he seeks to discover and use the laws of the universe, not only of inanimate nature but also of spiritual forces (Parrinder, 1965: 157). The medicine man believes that if his prescription is followed scrupulously, the results are certain. Hence, the saying in Emu that, "*Ogwu shikemeni ele nde*" (The medicine that is well cooked does not fail).

In Emu the *dibie* is saluted as "*Ogebunu Omenka*" (that is, the killer of ram; one who does good deeds) and they perform varied functions. He acts as a diviner, priest, herbalist and in some cases, a sorcerer. In carrying out these functions, he makes use of recipes which consist of appropriate mixture of herbs and other material objects as well as appropriate invocations and sacrifices. Thus, in curing or healing a mentally ill person for instance, the *dibie* uses medicinal herbs combined with invocation. The invocation is believed to give directions to the medicine and to trigger the powers contained in them.

Evans-Pritchard (1976: 428), while writing on the position of a medicine man in Azande society says, "I have not heard people speak highly of a man because he possesses medicines". It is the corollary of this view that is dominant in the Emu society. The *dibie*, by virtue of his strategic office in the society, is held in high esteem, despite the indifference exhibited by younger people due to the forces of modernization. In the olden days, the *dibie* was said to hold sway in political and spiritual affairs of the Emu society. He was consulted for solutions to knotty problems and his opinion was sought before important decisions were taken in the society (Enuadenu, 2003).

The *dibie's* profession is predominantly a male-vocation. Often of middle aged or older men, usually of affable and disposable nature. In the olden days, women did not practice as *dibie,* but this is changing in contemporary Emu society; there are now priestesses who combine their priestly duties with that of a *dibie*. Besides the professional *debie*, there are lay practitioners who seem to out-number the professional *dibie*. For clarity, lay-practitioner is used to refer to those possessing the knowledge and skill of some ritual medicines. These lay-practitioners cut across the young and old, students, civil servants, officers in the armed forces who practice medicine for their own self advancement.

It is expected that the professional medicine man, as a public practitioner, is competent in using his skills to solve the problems of his clients. Majority of the professional medicine men, who are untrained, often end up as quacks or frauds. This has made some observers of traditional medicine to be skeptical about medicinal claims; consequently they pass judgments on the practice of medicine and its practitioners in Emu. However, in the olden days of Emu, there was a section or lineage that worked as specialists, or professional mediciners. These professional medicine men were also religious specialist who can cause good or bad fortune by manipulating ritual processes. Arguing on the logical nexus that under-guards the ritual act of the medicine man among the Yoruba, Ade Dopamu states that for the medicine man,

> His logic rests on the belief that all objects possesses occult qualities, powers or forces which can be utilised by using those objects in which they reside. The objects in themselves are useless for ritual and medicinal purposes besides the occult power inherent in them. The occult power or forces radiate through nature and are hidden behind both animal and vegetable matters and can affect for good or ill whatever comes within their range, depending on the way man wants to utilize them (Dopamu, 1979: 508).

Although a competent medicine man (*dibie*) would have some knowledge of bad medicine, yet as a public practitioner, he would deal mainly with good medicines in order to maintain a good public image and retain an appreciable proportion of his clients. Evans-Pritchard writing on the conduct and accountability of medicine men, whom he designated as "witch doctors", says:

> Each witch-doctor acts on his own account, has his own practice, collects his own fees and generally speaking, is responsible to no one but himself in matters pertaining to professional conduct... He does not enter a guild in which all the members have socially important privileges and obligations for one another (1976: 209–222).

The above assertion is true of the Emu medicine men, who are not only scattered around the lineage groups and quarters of the community, but have no professional guild or association to oversee their conducts. His proficiency and good services can only be judged by his clients.

There are several forms of payment or financial transactions between a client and the medicine-man. For instance, the payment of a fee is the basis of the *panyilee Ogwu* (activating medicine) custom which demands that a client pays nominal fee to the medicine man for his work. This payment helps in "activating the medicine", since it is believed that without this token fee, the power to heal in the medicine would not be transmitted to the client. Another form of payment occurs to ensure the transfer of medicinal powers from the mediciner to a client. This transference of power is called *Ituye-ga-na-aka*. This literally means "throwing of sand into the hand". It is only when this symbolical action occurs that the efficacy of the medicine is guaranteed. Noting similarly, Malinowski (1970: 42) writes, "He (the medicine man) is repaid by small offerings immediately given and often incorporated into the ritual proceedings". A third form of payment in Emu is "*itie ife olili.*" This occurs as consultation fee; in essence, it shows that the clients is serious and has enlisted the services of the medicine man. This consultation fees is obligatory and it differs from one *dibie* to another. It could range from a bottle of local gin, kola-nuts and, or, money. When the client is a blood relation of the *dibie*, this payment may be waived. Fees could also be waived where the *dibie* has a special interest in the client. Evans-Pritchard long ago observed concerning the Azande Society that:

> If a man wishes medicine to be made on his behalf or to acquire possession of medicine, he has no difficulty in satisfying his desire. It is well known who possesses different medicine in a district, and these people are often kinsmen of or in some way socially linked with the man who requires their services (1976: 432).

Even when the requisite financial obligations are discharged, it is not certain that the sought power will be transferred. It is believed that a distant medicine man, i.e., not a close associate would never disclose all that he knows to his client or transfer all the power to his client. Thus, the medicine man who are kinsmen, relatives and lineage members are sought either to solve a problem or to help train another as a *dibie*.

5.2 The Training of a *Dibie*

There are different ways through which a person can become a *dibie* in Emu. It could be by calling from a deity or ancestor. According to my informant, the sign of a calling is perceived in numerous ways. It could be through physical illness or repeated dreams of somebody in the profession who is now dead. In the case of an illness, the person becomes afflicted with an unknown ailment which a *dibie* would divine to mean a call from an ancestral *dibie*. While in the dream, the person would see a dead relative, a *dibie*, calling the person to step into his shoes.

There are cases of people who understudy their parents or family members to learn the profession. Where this is the case, the father or a relative picks one of the children, and elects to train such favoured child. The training begins with the child accompanying the *dibie* father or relative as he performs his chores. Thus child learns by observing how the *dibie* father handles his clients and conducts his business. Gradually, the child is introduced to the different roots, barks, and leaves that make up ritual prescriptions. Over time duties are delegated to the student based on how quickly progress is made.

After this elementary stage, the learner is introduced to the core medicine; s\he is taught the fundamental elements that determine the efficacy of the different medicines, including their taboos, and injunctions. The learner, now acquainted with the instructor's repertoire, begins to practice basic medicine under supervision. If the student shows mastery of this stage and clients are happy with his\her success, s\he will move to the next stage and more duties are delegated to him\her. This process continues until the learner becomes qualified and in turn a full fledge *dibie*, who now can work independent of the instructor.

It is not every *dibie* apprentice that has the opportunity of learning from a *dibie*-father or relative. Majority of the *dibie* apprentice work their way through the learning process by understudying an established *dibie*. The education of such a person parallels that described for the person who understudies a parent of family member. They start from the rudimentary aspects till they become proficient. The difference between the father-son and apprentice-master relationships is that, the latter pays certain amount, either in terms of money, labor or services to his master.

The training of the apprentice could take a long time to complete. Normally, the training ends only when the apprentice had mastered the techniques of the different ritual prescriptions. As noted by lkenga-Metuh for the apprentice:

> He learns through observation and assisting their masters in how to handle people with different kinds of diseases and human problems. They master how to mix the different types of medicines, the different invocations, rituals and sacrifices that go with them and how to handle the different spiritual and human agencies of evil. He may be allowed to practice on his own, only after his character and professional competence have been certified by his master and he has been publicly initiated into the local guild of medicine men (1987: 224).

The initiation of an apprentice into the guild of medicine men is not practiced in Emu, since the *dibie* are independent and operate without any form of association or guild overseeing their craft. Each *dibie* is accountable only to their clientele. Instead of an initiation into the guild of practitioners, the Emu people organize a ceremony that is hosted by the master on behalf of the apprentice as a form of graduation party. At this ceremony, some of the *dibie* in that quarter or lineage group are invited to bless the new *dibie* and to wish him success in his career. This does not normally entail any elaborate ritual. The master simply announces publicly in the presence of other *dibie* from his quarters or lineage group that the apprentice has completed his training and his competence has been verified by him. From then on the apprentice is licensed to practice as a *dibie*.

5.2.1 The Functions of a *Dibie*

The duties of a *dibie* in Emu are diverse and varied. The *dibie* is at the same time a diviner, a healer, and a mediciner. According to Ikenga-Metuh (1987: 224):

> He is at once a physician, psychiatrist, a wonder-healer and a performer of rituals ... his main concern is with sickness, disease and misfortune... he can be called in to provide protective medicine for any form of misfortune just as he could be approached to prepare medicine to attract some fortunes, he can drive away evil spirits, track down witches and prepare antidote for sorcery. He could make medicine to guarantee abundant harvest, to prevent all sorts of pestilence, to cure infertility and to prevent constant child-deaths.

In carrying out his functions, the *dibie* does not perform on humanitarian basis in the sense of a philanthropist; rather he is a professional who makes a living off of his work. His office as a *dibie* is not a communal one. Nevertheless the *dibie* performs numerous functions that are strategic to the community's well-being. In carrying out his duties, the *debie* follows a pattern of diagnosis which makes him different from the Western medical doctor. Since he looks at a client's problem from a spiritual dimension, his solution entails spiritualism. This peculiar approach to clients' problems has been aptly described by Mbiti (1969: 169):

> The medicine man has therefore to discover the cause of the sickness, find out who the criminal is, diagnose the nature of the disease, apply the right treatment and supply a means of preventing the misfortune from occurring again... Thus, the medicine man applies both physical and spiritual treatments which assure the sufferer that all is and will be well. The medicine man is in effect both a doctor and a pastor to the sick person.

These are also spiritual problems which the medicine man could be called upon to solve in the community. One of such problems is the *Ogbanje* or the *abiku* syndrome. This is the belief that some children in the spirit world enter the wombs of their victims to be born only to die. The cycle of birth and death and rebirth torments the afflicted person. It would be up to the *dibie* to break this cycle and thus help the client to have a surviving child.

Lastly, it must be noted that the medicine man's activities are highly regarded by Emu people, unlike what Pritchard (1976: 26–40) suggested, they are not considered fraudulent or tricky. Their services have always been patronized by the rich and the poor, the educated and uneducated. The never ending patronage of the services of the *dibie* is a proof of their importance and perhaps a judgment of their trade. Consequently, Mbiti wrote:

> In short, the medicine men symbolize the hopes of society: hopes of good health, protection and security from evil forces, prosperity and good fortune and ritual cleansing when harm or impurities have been contracted. These men and women are intelligent and devoted to their work and those who are not simply do not prosper or get too far (Mbiti 1969: 170).

Although some *dibie* have been found to abuse their positions, this is not so for all, whatever abuses may be found in the activities of these practitioners are not enough to completely condemn their profession (Mbiti, 1975: 171).

5.3 Ritual Symbols and their Meanings in Emu Medicine

There is an abundance of symbols - in language, herbs and prescriptions within Emu ritual practices. In symbolism, the visible stands for the invisible, the material for the immaterial, the touchable for that which cannot be held or seized by sensory organs. Therefore, a symbol is a visible, tangible or audible representation of some conception or of some spiritual or intellectual reality (Kayode 1975: 34). Bell and Vogel describes symbol as, "something that stands for, represents, or denotes something else (not by exact resemblance) but by vague suggestion or by some conventional relation" (1963: 639). Symbol is, "a visible object or sound which stands for something which we already have direct knowledge of" (Bevan, 1962: 9). Different from the cited scholars, Radcliff-Brown considers symbols to be "whatever has meaning a symbol, the meaning being whatever is expressed by the symbol" (Radcliff-Brown, 1970: 69).

In the discussion of symbols and symbolic language, certain confusion had arisen with the usage of another word, "sign". This word is similar to but different from the word "symbol". According to Fawcett "Signs are denotative; they stand for or point to a specific object, event or person... signs are not intrinsic symbols; they have no built in resemblance with that which they signify" (Fawcett, 1970: 14). As obvious from these definitions, symbols are full of meanings which could be far removed from the immediate object or thing, while signs point to a specific thing or object and carries a message that is immediately discernible. Symbolic meanings are situational or circumstantial, which could differ greatly according to people, even among the same language family. The meaning of signs are not ambiguous, they indicate specific messages which enable the reader to identify its meaning (Wilson, 1971: 56).

In discussing the ritual symbolism and meaning of the Emu people's ritual practices, it is important to note following Turner, that, "when we talk about the meaning of a symbol, we must be careful to distinguish between at least three levels or fields of meaning" (Turner, 1970: 50). "One must first distinguish between information given by ritual specialists and information given by laymen; that is between esoteric and natural interpretations" Turner (1970: 12). The second is the operational meaning in the symbolic act. The symbol is not in itself considered separate from other components of the ritual proceedings, since the structure and composition help to complete the symbolic meaning. Another issue to explore into is the positional meaning of the symbol. This influences the kind of interpretation given to a symbol relative to another. In looking out for a symbolic meaning, one has to ask questions, such as, "what occasion brought about a ritual performance? For to a large extent, this occasion will not only shape the ritual performed, but that the end or purpose of such ritual will indicate the meaning of the symbols used" (Turner, 1965: 116). Against the presented background, the following sections examine the symbols used in medicinal rites in Emu as well as their meanings.

5.3.1 Medicine for Trade: *Ogwu Afia Okeawuli*

It would be recalled that the purpose of this medicine is to bring gain and profit to the user. The ritual for this medicine, *Ogwu afia okeawuli*, is performed by the *debie* himself and not the user. For these rites, the *dibie* collects the requisite ingredients, prominent among these ingredients are the head of a snake, white eagle feather, and the sand from the entrance of a market place. In Emu Community, the snake is known for the peculiar way it hunts for food. It stalks its victim and strikes swiftly. The victim is gripped by the mouth and swallowed by the snake. With this peculiar technique in hunting its prey, the snake is more at an advantage than other reptiles. To Emu people the eagle is a sacred bird that brings good fortune. It also stands for courage, dexterity and posture. The colour white symbolizes holiness, sacredness and prestige. Thus, the white eagle feather would bring honour to the user of the medicine for trade. The white eagle feather is also worn on the cap of some high ranking chiefs in the community. This feather, worn on another occasion by a titled man, would not only distinguish the person from the lower ranks of titled men of the community, but will indicate that the wearer is an important person, an achiever, a successful person of upright character. The feather on the cap could also signify a person that has been favoured or blessed by the divinities and ancestors. All these symbolic meanings are presumed to be transferred to the client through the use of medicine.

The *Eja onu ose*, which is "sand collected from the entrance to a market", is used in the ritual of *Ogwu afia okeawuli*. It plays an important role in achieving the final goal of the medicine. The earth or sand symbolizes the visible and the invisible forces, power and fertility. It also signifies the source of livelihood. In the people's tradition, it is believed that the market place does not only serve the living members of the community, but also the people of the spirit world. Thus, this earth that the spirit beings must have treaded on has an affinity with their persons. The spiritual person, who is the real self, which has an affinity with the sand, is summoned towards the stall of the user of the *Ogwu afia okeawuli*.

Another example of where the earth symbolises the unity of the living and the dead is *ituye ela na aka* (throwing or giving sand into the hand). It signifies spiritual power. This spiritual procedure is performed when the giver of the sand, a *dibie*, puts grains of sand into the hands of the recipient of the medicine to symbolize the transfer of authority to perform a medicine. During this process, the *dibie* repeats the phrase, "Let this medicine work". This action signifies the presence of the spiritual world to the transaction or transference of the medicinal power.

Elsewhere, *ituye ela na aka* is used to swear an oath as a proof of one's innocence. It is also used in the early morning prayers of *Igo ndi ke*', "the fellowship with the ancestors". During this fellowship, the *Ofo* stick is used to hit the ground in order to affirm a point or to ask for blessings. All these indicate to the Emu people that, the earth is alive with the ancestors as well as the spiritual powers that witness their daily activities. The incantations said over the pounding of the ingredients symbolize the accomplishment of the intended goal of the medicine. This is borne out of the belief that leaves, roots and barks are not only alive, but possess spiritual forces. When these forces are combined in the right proportion and prescription, their effectiveness is assured. In the light of the foregoing, the incantations during the pounding of the medicinal ingredients is performed to give direction to the medicine. It is believed that the latent spiritual forces present in each of these unified ingredients have spiritual ears and are awaiting instructions from the *dibie*. It is only at the time of pounding that the *dibie* must address these powers and instruct them with reference to their duties and functions.

5.3.2 Medicine for Love: *Ogwu Isorlu obe Mmalu*

This medicine, as already introduced, is used by an intended lover to attract a spouse or love interest even against their will. Some of the prominent items that are included in the preparation that convey meaning are the leaves that sprout where red ants cluster, the placenta of a goat, and the feather of a parrot. These items are believed to be the essential ingredients, without which the ritual will fail. The red ants signify aggressiveness, stubbornness, and determination. The leaves that sprout where the red ants cluster indicate strength, ability to conquer amidst difficulties and oppositions. Thus, the leaves symbolise the triumph of the user over the unwilling and unbending strong will of the love interest that is sought. The symbolism of the placenta of a goat has been noted by Mbiti for the Gikuyu birth and childhood rituals. According to Mbiti (1975: 113), "the placenta and the umbilical cord are the symbols of a child's attachment to the mother, to womanhood". The placenta, therefore, symbolises a physical and spiritual attachment of a child to the mother. This attachment is lifelong. Similarly, the placenta of a goat in this medicine signifies the kind of close relationship that would exist between the user of the medicine and the intended victim. It is presumed that since the close relationship has taken place spiritually, it must also exist in the physical.

The parrot is peculiar among the other birds for certain reasons. The Emu people believe that the bird is one of the most attentive listeners; it is quick, smart and can imitate a voice or sound. The parrot also has the ability to survive under unfavourable conditions and can function as a messenger that bears accurate tales for the spirits. The parrot's feather in this medicine therefore symbolises the target's ability to grasp and imitate, by obeying the commands or request of the user. These commands must be spoken to the hearing of the target. The verbal expression of the user's intentions to the target is a vital part of this rite without it the ritual procedure is incomplete.

Further, just as the feather on the cap of a chief serves to distinguish his\her status, the parrot's feather distinguishes the user's request in the midst of other advances from other suitors. Hence, the phrase in the incantation that says, "*efeluche ekwe omali ni ikpo ebuba*" (The parrot's feather is not difficult to be identified in the midst of other feathers). Lastly, the *nzu* (white chalk), which is sprinkled on the pounded ingredients signifies sacredness, holiness and prestige. The sprinkling of the *nzu* symbolises a sacred sealing of the medicine, that is the "amen" or "so shall it be"

5.3.3 Medicine to aid Memory: *Ogwu Akonuche*

According to Chukwudi Odalue (1990), *ogwu akonuche* is used to aid the retention of information. It helps the user to remember all that s\he has heard and understood. In the ritual processes, as discussed in Chapter Three, three of the ingredients in preparation are: a mouse, a small fish, and alligator pepper. These items are the most important of the ingredients in this medicine. Among the Emu people, the mouse is considered one of the smallest but least forgetful animals in the animal kingdom. It is said that once the mouse had set a task for itself, it always remembers to execute it. It does not matter how enormous the task might be. Thus, it symbolizes an unfailing memory, alertness, and wisdom to recount what one has committed to memory.

The fish is ever present in the water and never escapes the fisherman's trap. Thus, it is used to symbolize constancy, strength and accuracy. These qualities by transference are imputed to the user. The alligator pepper is traditionally never absent neither is far from the kolanut. Its peppery flavour can never go unnoticed in the mouth. It, therefore, symbolizes recognition, remembrance and continuity. In the ritual of *Ogwu akonuche*, the spiritual forces inherent in the ritual medicine must be activated when it is to be used. To do this, the user licks the medicinal paste and recites the incantation provided by the dibie. With these works, the power within the medicine are activated and sent forth.

5.3.4 Medicine to Ward off Rain: *Ogwu Ifemmili*

Idonor lsakpa (1990) explains that this medicinal rite is used to ward off rainfalls that are disruptive to festive and ceremonial occasions. Among the various items used for the ritual are red ants and the leaves of the oil bean tree. In the Emu community, red ants are known for their ability to spread out rapidly to reform a colony when disturbed. Thus, the ants symbolise order, rapidity, willingness to change positions and swiftness. The ants also represent a spiritual order of change with less obstruction. The red ants differ from other ants like the giant black ants, in the sense that when the giant black ants are disturbed, they do not become aggressive or stubborn. The symbolism of the leaves of the oil bean tree is the opposite of that of the red ants.

The leaves of the oil bean tree cannot be used to wrap or store food. These leaves are scattered on the ground symbolising disunity, disharmony, disorderliness and inability to stay together. As noted, the ingredients are tied together with the right proportion of other ingredients and hung on top of a low burning fire to produce cloud of smoke. Thus the symbolic power of these ingredients is transferred to the rain cloud. As Wilson (1971: 35) pointed out, "Clouds of smoke do not only symbolise rain, but also cause rain".

In the incantations for this ritual, the words give power and direction to the medicinal ingredients. The words in the incantation that says, "The *ichite* leaves can never grow on dead wood" describes the orderliness of nature and the impossibility of nature to go against its natural rhythm. *Emu* people believe that controlling the rain, for those who know how, is a natural process. Since the *ichite* leaves cannot grow on dead wood, it is believed that the rain cloud can never refuse to move. It must obey the medicine man's command.

5.4 Ritual Symbolism in Therapeutic Medicines

5.4.1 Medicine to Cure Belly Ache: Ogwu Efo Olinwa

According to our informant, Oliver Abanum, one of the subjects, the goal of this medicinal rite is to cure belly aches. In the ritual procedure of *Ogwu efo olinwa,* there are two ingredients that carry symbolic meanings. These are the *uda*, a spice, and the native white chalk, *nzu*. The *uda* may symbolise peace or trouble, depending on the circumstance of use. The symbolism of the *nzu* has already been explained, it represents sacredness, power, seal, or agreement in the spiritual realm. The important stage of this particular rite is in *ipayi lee ogwu*, "the activation of medicine." This is the ritual custom where the client pays the *dibie* a token fee, as part of the ritual processes of making the medicine work. This aspect of the ritual represents the people's belief that you have to give something to possess anything of value. It is more so when acquiring spiritual powers. With this token, it becomes obligatory to the *debie* to acquiesce to clients' demand even if such is against his wishes.

5.4.2 Medicine to Cure Venereal Diseases: *Ogwu Emo Uku Igbele*

This is another therapeutic medicine used to cure venereal disease and prevent miscarriages. In the ritual proceedings for this rite, the *dibie* gathers appropriate ingredients that are pounded to produce the medicine. Prominent among these ingredients are the root of a coconut tree, the root of a lime tree, and the root of a kolanut tree. The root of the coconut tree symbolises energy, prosperity and fertility. In the olden days, the coconut fruit is eaten as food alone or mixed with other foods. The water from the coconut is sweet and serves as drink to refresh the body. The lime root signifies strength and curative power of the divine. The lime tree symbolises mystical powers that are active in all the properties: roots, bark, leaves and fruit. Its presence in medicinal ritual indicates the presence of the mystical curative power of the spiritual world.

The root of the kola nut tree denotes abundant life, the physical and spiritual abundance of life. Thus, it is believed since it stands for life, it will not co-exist with sickness or things that threaten life. Also, the kolanut tree symbolises sacredness and holiness in the community. The kolanut can never be used for poison or destructive purposes; it is the symbol of God's presence, goodness, wellbeing and happiness. Therefore, anything that threatens these characteristics, ultimately threatens the divine. The cowries tied around the neck of the bottle with the medicinal substance indicates the presence of the divine, sanctity, and spiritual sanction. According to my informant, without these cowries, the spiritual forces active in the medicine will dissipate after the time allotted for its operation has expired (Oliver Abanurn, 1990).

5.4.3 Medicine to Keep a Dying Man Awake: *Mmuo ni Mmalu afu enya*

According to Nwabefa, my informant, this particular ritual medicine is used to keep a dying man alive and conscious until all arrangements pertaining to his estate has been concluded. This medicine can sustain such a man for a short period of time. The symbolism involved in this preparation cannot be determined by isolating single ingredients and examining them for meaning, as has been done for other ritual medicines that have been discussed thus far. The goal of the medicine is to severe contacts between the man and the pending spiritual world. The ritual ingredients consist of leaves, roots, gun powder and local white chalk (*nzu*).

The leaves and the roots which must not be separated symbolises the existence and source of strength. It is believed that death occurs when the original source of strength (breath) is cut off spiritually. This is why the root, together with the leaves, which must be in one whole are used for medicinal preparation. The gun powder symbolises a break, a blackout on the spiritual world. It shuts out the physical world from the spiritual world, making it temporarily invisible to the spiritual world. This means that, the personification of death will be blind and unable to deliver the message of death to the victim. Lastly, the use of local white chalk indicates a seal, a sacred bond on the part of spiritual forces to keep to the goals of the ritual, which thus guarantees the efficacy of the medicine.

5.4.4 Medicine to Cure the Mentally Ill: *Ogwu Enya Enu*

The purpose of this medicinal ritual is to cure mental illness. The mentally ill person must not be a chronic case, i.e., a person who had been mad for a long time. This medicine reverses to normalcy somebody who recently became mentally ill. There are symbolisms in some of the core ingredients of this medicine which include: black local soap, leaves from a grave, sand from a burial ground, grass obtained close to a well, and, the liquid from a snail water. There are taboos associated with collecting these items. For instance, when collecting the sand, one must close his eyes before scooping some sand into his hand, so also with the grass that grows beside a well. The *dibie* must not be seen by anyone when collecting these items. The black soap symbolizes spiritual cleansing of the body from all evil forces. Since the colour black symbolizes evil, so it is believed that the black soap would wash away the spiritual evil that might be causing the mental condition of the person. The leaves from the grave of a dead person symbolize the active presence of the spirit world which is believed to be responsible for what goes on in the visible, physical world. Among the people of Emu, it is a tradition to make a grave for only those that died 'a good death'. Those who died 'a bad death', usually as a result of evil deeds, are buried in, or thrown into, the bad bush.

The earth represents the collective presence of the visible and invisible powers. The earth is believed to be alive with powers, in this case it represent the spiritual world of the dead which are believed to inhabit the earth. The grass from around a well symbolizes the source of being, life and health. The well in the community is the main source of water for domestic purposes. It is a meeting point for everybody, since each makes daily trip to it for water. Therefore, the grass connects with health, life and the source of being. The liquid of a snail symbolizes purity, impotence, and powerlessness in the visible and invisible realm. The liquid stagnates, nullifies and reduces the efficacy of negative spiritual powers that comes in contact with it. The liquid from a snail nullifies all negative forces and thus activates the curative powers of the other ingredients in the medicine.

Writing on the symbolism of African people Mbiti (1969: 27) says, the invisible world is symbolized or manifested by these visible and concrete phenomena and objects of nature. The invisible world presses hard upon the visible: one speaks of the other, and the African people 'see' the invisible universe when they look at, hear or feel the visible and tangible world. This is one of the fundamental heritages of African people. Thus, the black soap would clean away the spiritual evil, the leaves from the grave world, through the goodness of the spirits and ancestors, will cure the mental illness, the sand will bring in the invisible world to sanction the purpose of the ritual, the leaves from the well will restore normalcy and good health and the liquid of the snail will counteract all negative forces.

5.5 Ritual Symbols in Protective Medicines

Under this category are rituals performed to either ward off evil forces or protect an individual from destructive medicines. These set of medicines contain several symbols, they are described in the following subsections.

5.5.1 Protective Medicine against Poison: *Aju Ogwu*

This medicinal ritual is aimed at protecting the user from poison, be it physical or spiritual poisons. The basic ingredients of the ritual are eggs, termites, and young palm frond. These items carry in them meanings that are beyond the physical properties. The egg symbolizes life, rebirth, freshness and coolness. This essence of egg, which is summed up in life itself, must revolt or counter anything that threatens life and general well-being. Thus, the egg aids the medicine by re-affirming life, bringing freshness and vitality to oppose any poison. The termite symbolizes strength, steadiness, and impregnability. This spiritual essence which the termite symbolizes is passed on to the ritual medicinal process. Through their strength and sturdiness, they are able to build an impregnable colony which protects them from their enemies and vagaries of nature. Thus, destructive medicine or poison will not be able to penetrate the strength, hardness and stiff barrier which the termite symbolizes. The bunch of young palm fronds symbolizes the presence of the spiritual world and their potent power. Sometimes, the young palm frond indicates the presence of the harbinger of death or evil-forces. This is so when it is used in connection with death. As Basden (1938: 275) had recorded among the Ibos:

> Before digging the grave, a bunch of young palm-leaves (*mmu*) is taken. A young man beats the ground with these, crying, as he does so, he says let the old dead body depart because a new (dead) body has come.

With the harbinger of death duly represented by the symbolism of the young palm frond, the user of this medicine is believed to be protected from any form of death by poisoning. Consequently, this agreement is sealed with the sprinkling of local white chalk, thereby making poison powerless when used against the person protected by *aju ogwu*.

5.5.2 Medicine against Destructive Medicine: Ogwu Nkpokwa

According to Abanum my informant, this particular medicine is used against general attacks from destructive medicine. It protects the user from sorcerers, witches, and from all evil intentions. In this ritual, some of the important items are the barks of *iroko* tree, oil bean tree, the head of an animal and *neoboldia* leaves tree. The *iroko* tree in the community is the biggest and the strongest among trees. It is believed to be full of life, hence its longevity. Its wood is a comfortable abode for spirits who are present in the community. Thus, the bark of the *iroko* tree stands for the aforementioned qualities. The *iroko* tree also symbolizes the primordial existence of the first ancestors of the community. It was this tree that give shelter and security to the first ancestors (*olor ne emu*) of the community. Therefore, the symbolism is that the *iroko* tree will not allow destructive and evil medicine to harm the user of *ogwu nkpokwa* since the bark of the iroko tree represents the presence of these protective spirits in the ritual procedures.

The oil bean tree could be likened to the Detarium Senegalese tree from which the *ofo* stick is made. According to Edmund Ilogu:

> It is believed that *Chukwu* (the Great God) purposely created this tree to be sacred and by the manner its branches fall off unbroken, he (*Chukwu*) symbolizes the way families grow up and establish new extended families or lineage (1974: 18).

The difference between the symbol of the Detarium Senegalese tree and the oil bean tree is that, the latter symbolizes the manner in which destructive and evil medicine fall off in tiny bits without reaching its target. The bark of the oil bean tree symbolizes frustration and inaccessibility. Therefore, in the context of *Ogwu nkpokwa,* this symbolism implies that repeated attacks against the user of the medicine will only end in frustration.

The *neoboldja* tree symbolizes the presence of the sacred and at times the divine. This tree is planted when a new house is under construction and serves as the temple of the Supreme Being in every village and compound. At the foot of the tree the people worshipped and prayed to the Supreme Being. The presence of the bark of the *neoboldia* tree among the items in the ritual process means that the divine, the ancestors and *Chukwu* (God), are called in to protect the user of *Ogwu nkpokwa* against all known and unknown forces.

The head of the animal symbolizes the spiritual essence of the user. Consequently, it is believed that the *iroko* bark will strengthen it, the bark of oil bean tree will frustrate whatever plot is directed against it through destructive and evil medicine. The bark of the *neobolja* tree will see to it that the user is protected against all forms of attacks. Finally, in the ritual, the local white chalk, *nzu*, as used in most medicinal rituals, provides blessings.

5.5.3 Medicine to Prevent Evil Occurrence: *Njo Puazu*

As the name of the medicine implies, its user will always elude troubles and evils. The prominent items used in preparation of the medicine are leaves, broomsticks, and the horn of an antelope. First, the leave which while hanging on its branch is turned towards the city symbolizes the eyes with gaze to the world. Since the road represents the world of all those coming in or going out, it is thought that something that is keeping an eye on the road will surely be able to see what comes in and goes out. Thus, with the leaves' ability to see, it will readily inform the user of the medicine of any impending evil. This information is transmitted to the user as premonition.

The broomstick symbolizes clearance, the removal of evil. It also indicates the triumph of good over evil. Since the broom is never used to sweep away goods, but dirt and rubbish, so also the ill that is intended to the user of *njo puazu* medicine will always be cleared away from him\her. The horn of an antelope symbolizes safety and invincibility. Evil in the community is personified as somebody who from time to time seeks to harm its victims or cause them misfortune. Therefore, the antelope which, in the context of this ritual represents the user of *njo puazu,* will be empowered to hasten away from evil. It is also believed that the horn of an antelope in the ritual will help the user become invincible, unreachable and therefore evil will not be able to seek him out for harm.

5.5.4 Medicine for Cutlass and Knife Protection: *Ogwu Mma*

This medicinal ritual is performed to safeguard the user from cutlass and knife attacks such that when attacked, these weapons will leave no wounds. Items such as the nest of soldier ants, the shells of a porcupine, snail, and tortoise are used in the preparation of this ritual medicine. In the symbolism of these items lies the idea of opposing or antithetical forces of the biting powers of the soldier ants and the protective powers of animal shells. The shell of the porcupine indicates power, impregnability, hardness and toughness. It symbolizes the protective power which is physically and spiritually inherent in these shells. Just as the stings of the ants are ineffective against the shell of the porcupine, the cutlass and knife will be weak against the protective shield that is now transferred to the user by the medicine.

Finally, it must be stated that these symbolic meanings are not just fancies of the *dibie* whom the skeptic will be quick to represent as skilful in fraud and trickery. It seems that it is against this background that Parrinder (1969: 157) has generalized that many medicines are selected because of some observed or fancied resemblance to the illness. A spotted leaf may be thought to be a good remedy for spotted skin and a sharp quill ought to act as protection against enemies of the soul. Such misunderstanding of the symbolic meanings of African ritual practices has led Mbiti (1975: 57) to suggest that:

> It is unfortunate that foreign writers through great ignorance, having failed to understand this deep Religious insight of our people; and have often either ridiculed it or naively presented it as "nature worship" or "animism". Traditional African societies have been neither deaf nor blind to the spiritual dimensions of existence which is so deep, so rich and so beautiful.

5.5.5 Medicine for Gunshot Protection: *Ogwu Egbe Ufie*

This particular medicine is used to protect the user from gunshot and sharp objects. In the ritual procedure, like all protective medicine, different items form the list of ingredients. However, basic to the ritual are coco-yam and gun cartridge. In the community, the coco-yam plant is believed to possess active spiritual powers that are dangerous to any evil forces. The evil force must have to retreat or gets destroyed when it comes in contact with the coco-yam plant. It is this belief among the Emu people that gave rise to the planting of coco-yam near or around their houses. It is thought that with the plant around their houses, evil forces like the witches can never get through to them. Thus, the coco-yam symbolizes a barrier, obstacle, and protective shield that cannot be surmounted by a negative spiritual power; as such the user is shielded from gunshots. It is believed that the bullet coming out of a gun is evil and destructive; therefore, it will not be able to penetrate the effective protective barrier which the coco-yam plant symbolizes (Chukwukuni 1990). The cartridge symbolizes the evil, destructive force of the gun. The presence of the cartridge in the ritual procedure indicates the capture, subjugation of the particular evil that could injure the user.

5.6 Ritual Symbols and their meanings in Destructive Medicines

Medicine rituals for destructive purposes are not as commonly practiced as productive and protective medicine. This is not to suggest that, there are no medicinal rituals for destructive ends. As a matter of fact, their rituals are as elaborate and full of symbolic meaning as in protective medicine.

5.6.1 Medicine to 'Shoot' Poison: *Ogwu Igba Nkpa*

Ogwu igba nkpa is used mainly to send poisonous substance, objects, and materials into the body of a victim. These poisonous materials shot into the body, will in time, lead to the death of the victim, except it is not removed. In the ritual procedure, the *dibie,* who performs the medicine, collects amongst other ingredients a dead millipede, a toad, a chameleon, a needle, and alligator pepper. The millipede is believed to create and attract conditions favourable for evil forces to launch attack on its victim. Usually, Emu people do not kill a millipede when it crawls into the house; it is carefully picked up and thrown outside. It is thought that its death will bring evil into such a home. The toad symbolizes the messenger of death, wretchedness, and bad fortune. It is believed that the toad bears these evil messages to a victim. The toad never carries good fortune to a victim; it is solely associated with evil forces.

The chameleon symbolizes paralysis and complete destruction. The chameleon, like the toad and millipede, can never be used for protective or curative purposes. Their presence constitute bad omen, the presence of evil, thus they are carefully avoided. The needle symbolizes pain, and ability to injure its victim. Although, the needle could be used for other ritual purposes, but in this ritual, it serves the purpose of causing pains to its victim. When the needle is used in the ritual of *Ogwu igba nkpa,* it is believed that it will weaken the victim and ultimately kill the victim. It is, therefore believed that with the millipede inviting and creating conducive atmosphere for attack against its victim, and the toad effectively carrying destructive messages, the chameleon destroying and paralyzing the targeted victim, and with the pain coming from the needle, the intended target will be fatally harmed by this medicine.

From the aforementioned instances, it is apparent that the people's medicinal rituals are full of symbolism. Some of the symbolic meanings of the items cannot be fully grasped when considered independent of the whole items that constitute the ingredients of the ritual practice. It has been observed that symbols do not denote things which are already understood, but attempt to push forward the frontiers of knowledge and to grasp the reality of things, the real nature of life. These symbols push beyond the frontiers of empirical objectivity and seek a subjective approbation of the transcendent (Fawcett 1970: 20). In their selection of symbols, the people of Emu are not contented with the mere handling of these physical things but are endowed with a passion for knowledge of the meaning which lies behind them.

The opinions of foreign observers of medicinal rituals, that consider these rites as inadequate and irrelevant, must not be taken seriously. As Radcliff-Brown (1952: 44) had erroneously generalized when commenting on the totemic rites of an Australian tribe that:

> The ostensible purpose of these rites as stated by the nature is to renew or maintain some part of nature such as, specie of animal or plant, a rainy or hot or cold weather. With reference to this purpose we have to say that from our point of view the natures are mistaken, that the rites do not actually do what they are believed to do. The rain making ceremony does not actually bring rain. In so far as the rites are performed for a purpose they are futile, based on erroneous belief.

Emu people do not see their ritual practices as false and meaningless. These rites, as Otubanjo has also noted, are symbolic representation of some ideas of beliefs (Otubanjo, 1987: 33).

Chapter Six: Continuity and Change in Emu World View

This chapter is a description of the religious beliefs and ritual practices of the Emu people within the contemporary context and the change effected. The advent of Christianity in Emu Community was heralded by the Anglican Church, which spread from Ewurie-Aradhe in Isokoland. According to Iwegbue, the Anglican Church was introduced into Emu by Mr. Onu Adanu, who was frustrated by the constant death of his children. He heard about the miraculous activities of the new religion; how a lot of sick people who had joined the new faith had been healed, how the converts had been delivered from their troubles; how those in bondage, i.e., *osu* were freed, how the powers of witchcraft and sorcery had been neutralized, and how the barren received children. He abandoned his indigenous religion and travelled with his household to Ewurie-Aradhe to accept the Christian faith. Thus, Mr. Onu and his household became the earliest nucleus of Anglican community in Emu (Iwegbue, 1981: 7).

Catholicism is also found in Emu, it spread to Emu from the neighbouring Abbi Town. Madam Juliana Ogbogo, a traveller and trader who had long loathed some aspects of the traditional religion and culture which she considered to be at variance with her ideals in life, took to the new religion at Abbi. She returned to Emu with her new found faith and encouraged everyone in her household and lineage to join. Thus, like Onu Adanu, Ogbogo and her household were the pioneers of the Catholic faith in Emu (according to Enyabine interviewed 1988).

At their onset, Emu people received the new religion and co-operated with its missionaries. They believed that the Christian faith was not antagonistic to their indigenous religion and that the worship of the "white-man's god" could be carried on alongside their traditional religion. The missionaries easily won the heart of the members of the community. They executed building projects such as churches and schools. By 1927, Church and school were already established in Emu. The early Christians in Emu consisted of those that abandoned their traditional religion (Okoligwe, 1987).

The new form of education introduced by the missionaries in Emu intoxicated the people like new wine. The ability to read and write was a new craze that helped to attract those who yearned to be like the white-man. In addition to this, the benefits of the white-man's education was clearly visible in the community. Education quickly transformed the occupational structure of the Emu Community. Those that went early to *Uno* School (mission school) and had become proficient in the white-man's language assumed new positions of influence. Chief Tom Edengulu Owete and G. Iwegbue early beneficiaries of this education became representatives and spokesmen of the people. Thus, there arose among the people, great envy and desire to be like their fellowmen with these new status. This ambition could only be met through the mission school and the church, the only available educational centres at that time. Consequently, a good number of the people went to the church, to learn to read and write and to speak the white-man's language. Education was augmented with the teachings from the Bible, the effect of which was to cause a break with their indigenous religion.

However, there were instances when the people changed their religion based on admiration or spiritual satisfaction. Using Dopamu's words to describe Emu people's condition at this time, a person who has wallowed for years under a particular problem would not hesitate to embrace a religion that solves this problem for him (Dopamu, 1979: 112–113). The persistent attack by the missionaries on the people's long held beliefs, to some extent, caused some of them to break away from some aspects of their indigenous religion and converted to Christianity. For some others who believe that Christianity could not be reconciled with traditional values, they preferred to disobey the laws of the traditional deities and violate the taboos of the land.

The Christian community in Emu was a close knit society of converts who were each other's brother's keeper. In the pursuit of their beliefs, they flagrantly violated all the food taboos and the traditional *eke* day, a "day of rest"; they brought out their charms and ritual symbols and burnt them and they made songs that ridiculed the *dibie's* powers (lwegbue 1987). The emergence of plurality of religious beliefs and values in Emu triggered the start of a rapid social change similar to that which has been going on in neighboring Igboland. Christians challenged Igbo (Emu) traditional beliefs as well as such social control methods like divination and consultation of oracles (Ilogu, 1974: 88).

This notwithstanding, the belief in witchcraft and sorcery continued unabated in Emu even up to this time. While many Christian converts no longer believe that either the good medicine or bad medicine can have any effect on them, some others still dread sorcerers and consequently make use of Holy Water and other symbols of Christianity to protect themselves. As Christianity held sway in the Emu community, it became common for people to confess to owning bad medicine and renouncing them unlike the earlier times, as such there was a remarkable reduction in the practice of bad medicine. The situation was different from the pre-colonial times when social miscreants and misfits were disposed of with the aid of bad medicine. Also, because of the impact of Christianity, land cases among the Emu people no longer result in the use of potent bad medicine. Instead, people sought justice first through the traditional judicial system of the council of elders, and if unsatisfied with the outcome, they resorted to the law courts. Evidently, the institution of colonialism, western education and the effective proselytizing activities of the missionaries not only transformed the Emu community, it equally strengthened their skepticism about their indigenous religion.

The transformation in Emu due to new religion led to the erosion of the prestige and esteem of the *debie*. Central to this was the introduction by the colonial government of a new form of health services called the "dispensary". This health system was more effective and cheaper compared to the elaborate ritual of the indigenous health care system. The activities of the *dibie* in some quarters of the community got upended. Consequently, the reverence and veneration of the various Emu deities ebbed drastically.

6.1 Change and Continuity in the Beliefs and Rituals concerning *Olor*

The name *Olonemu* was derived from *Olor* and *Emu*. Olor was the husband of Emu. According to oral tradition the Oba of Benin Kingdom had vowed to possess Emu from Olor. For this reason Olor decided to flee with his wife from Benin Kingdom. As they ran away from the Benin Kingdom, they came to a big river close to the present day Agbor Kingdom. The couple encountered difficulties and found it impossible to cross the big river. They had no canoe and pursuing them were the people sent by the Oba to bring the woman back to Benin. After some time of depression, two alligators (male and female) came out of the river and carried Olor and Emu across the river to the other side. The male alligator carried Olor, while the female alligator carried Emu. When the people pursuing them got to the bank of the river they did not find them. Unsatisfied at this, they crossed the river with canoes, hoping they would catch up with the couple. Unfortunately, they did not find any footprints, because a bird called *Okolobise*, had scratched off the footprints of Emu and Olor. Disappointedly, they went back to the Oba of Benin without Emu.

Olor is therefore worshipped by the people of Emu till today. According to the interviewee, "it is here in my house, as the head of the village (*Okpala*). The female is here in my house and the male is in the house of the other village head (*Okpala-Uku*), because he is older and also the overall clan head". There is a stream that is called *Olor*. That stream is named after the shrine and it is the boundary between Abbi Community and Emu. The stream belongs to Emu Community. *Olor* is a god of the land and it is believed that it will punish anyone that violates its injunctions. To determine if there has been violations against *Olor*, a person has to consult the oracle or it will be revealed to the person in the dream. Then, if it is confirmed that the person has offended *Olor*, s\he will offer the appropriate sacrifice for cleansing. The substance of sacrifice for cleansing consists in four chicks (two for the female *Olor* and two for the male *Olor*), a hen, one *Atuma,* fish, one *Olili,* fish. The afore-listed objects taken to the *Okpala-Uku*'s palace where the sacrifice is performed. If it the person who committed infractions against Olor has been struck with illness by Olor, the following ingredients are offered as sacrifice on behalf of the sick person: eight pieces of plantain, ten tubers of yam, a bottle of palm oil, salt, potash (*Akeu*), eight pieces of kolanut and pepper. All the ingredients are taken to *Obodo-Uku* where *Olor* first lived and there they are cooked. Nothing that is taken to *Obodo-Uku* is brought back to Emu. The leftovers are thrown away. This practise has continued till today.

However, during a normal worship of *Olor*, the following items are used: yam, palm oil, kolanut, native chalk (*Nzu*), white cloth. The yam is dried then pounded into powder which is divided into two parts. One part is mixed with little oil and the other part is left in the powdered form. The pieces of the kolanut are thrown with their faces upwards before the shrine, so also the powdered yam (yam flour). During the worship of *Olor* and or offering of sacrifice, the chief priest wears a special costume. The bag of *Olor* is taken from the palace of the *Okpala* and the priest hangs it on his left hand. He moves from there to the palace of the *Okpala-Uku*, where the preparations are arranged. Women are forbidden to pass by the left hand of the priest when he is going for worship or to offer sacrifice to *Olor*. As soon as the priest comes out, any woman that sees him with the bag hanging on his right shoulder must cross to the other side of the road. These effects have strangely defied time. There are several prohibitions and rules that are peculiar to *Olor*. A woman having her period must not walk past the shrine of Olor. Violation will cause the flow of her menstrual period to cease. To avoid this, a separate road is provided for menstruating women.

However, the woman that has been afflicted by the god can be cured if the god is appeased. To do this, one white cock is required of her. This is used to run gently through her body, from head to toe. The cock is then thrown alive into the shrine. The prohibitions of *Olor* is that her children (*Emu* people) should not kill or stay to watch the killing of an alligator (*oba, nneemu*). This same prohibition applies to the bird called *Okolo-bise*. If a son or daughter of *Emu* origin eats any of these unknowingly, *Olor* will reveal the offence to the person in a dream. The person is then expected to come home for the necessary remedial action "if he is wise". Sometimes, one could see the alligator tied up for sale in the market, but should not buy it. However, such a person is expected to return to the village and perform the sacrifice required for cleansing. If one intentionally eats either the alligator or the bird his or her body will swell up as punishment. Also, it is believed that if someone sees an alligator tied up and the person sings songs of praises to the tied alligator, the alligator will cheer up and will show its happiness by jumping up and down and prancing around. The person who saw the tied-up alligator will endeavor for it to be untied. It is believed that *Olor* is the god of protection. According to Chief B. Enyabegwu, "if people try to attack any *Emu* man anywhere, he will escape mysteriously, without anyone noticing him. This is made possible by *Olonemu* who makes the Emu person invisible to his\her attackers. It is this protection that gave rise to the saying, "*Olonemu gbo ogu, onye Emu ona*" (the god, *Olor*, will always separate a fight for an *Emu* man to escape)". In the recent past Ogume, a neighboring community warred with Emu. During the war, Emu men were made invisible to *Ogume* men. Based on this story, the interviewee maintained that *Olor* is still very active irrespective of the influence of Christianity. He further stated that, if a person violates any of the prohibitions of *Olor*, despite being a Christian, the person must surely come to appease *Olor* or die. However, George Dakwa, another informant, asserted that there has been less patronage and sacrifice to *Olor*.

6.2 Continuity and Change in the Beliefs and Rituals Concerning *Nze*

It should be recalled that among the people of Emu *Nze* is the god of war and the custodian of mental health. Oral tradition holds that after the legendary Obumkpomkpo killed *Ubejiagana*, a mermaid (see chapter 2), he brought its head to *Emu-Unor*, where his father, lyasele, received him. Iyasele, who is from Ajonogu clan, asked his friend to take Obumkpomkpo to his home to stay with him. A hut was erected outside Ogbolum's house, where Obumkpomkpo kept his bag containing the head of Ubeiagana and the machete (*Ogbodo*), with which he had cut off the head. Obumkpomkpo called the content of his bag *Nze*. He went on to explain to Ogbolum the taboos of this new god and how to serve it. It is in this context that Ogbolum assumed the position of the priest of *Nze* in Emu. In the course of worshipping and serving, the chief priest and the people from Ogbolum started making monetary gains, by charging high fees. The people of the Ajonogu clan, on seeing the material benefits of being the custodian of the *Nze* shrine, started making claims over it. In their claim, they stressed that the man that brought *Nze* was originally from Ajonogu and as such it should be returned to Ajonogu. However, the Ogbolum clan refused to hand *Nze* back to them. This refusal made the Ajonogu clan to prepare their own *Nze*. As a result there are now two *Nze* shrines in Emu Community, the one at Ogbolum and the other at Ajonogu.

It is believed that the chief priest of *Nze* (called *Oyiwa*) must come from Ogbolum clan, the appointment therefore, is not on a rotational basis. According to Chief Patrick Enuademu, if a person who was meant to be a family chief priest declined to do so on the grounds of his Christian faith, the next elderly man in the family will become the chief priest (Enuademu, 2003). The interviewee went on to say that not too long ago the members of Ajonogu Street claimed that they were to produce the chief priest of *Nze*. This agitation was as a result of a prior incident. At that time, some Emu people living in Lagos sent one the sum of Naira Fifty Kobo (₦ 1.50) to appease *Nze*. Unfortunately, this appeasement was not made and the problem plaguing the Emu people in Lagos continued. Worried, the Emu people in Lagos wrote to find out why the money was not utilized for the purpose it was sent, and requested for a refund. They, in their letter stated clearly that the money was given to Chief Iwema, the then *Onotu-Ukwu* (head of the clan chiefs), who hailed from Etevie Street. All the other chiefs in amazement trooped went to the *Onotu-Ukwu* to find out what really happened. The *Onotu-Ukwu*, in order to cover up the disgrace, feigned anger and in the bid to save face went to Ajonogu quarters and incited the people to demand for the position of the chief priest of *Nze*. The *Onotu-Ukwu* told the people of Ajonogu that they were the rightful quarter to produce the *Oyiwa*, since they were meant to be the custodian of *Nze*. Based on the Ajonogu quarters began to agitate for the right to field the *Oyiwa*.

Robert Baum (1999: 119) writing on the Diola Religion and Society in pre-colonial Senegambia argued that the introduction of *Hupila Kudjenk* was closely associated with the increasing wealth of those who raided or sold captives. When asked why a new form of *Hupila* was adopted, informants frequently cited the desire to display their new wealth in a more socially acceptable way. Analogous experience was recorded during the institutionalisation of the *Nze* at Ajonogu. They of the Ajonogu quarters, according to the interviewee, made it mandatory that anyone coming to worship should come to Ajonogu.

Every five years, the five communities that make up Emu gather to worship the *Nze* at Ogbolum. One of the five communities is chosen to produce the ram to be used for the worship of *Nze*. This is done in a rotational basis every five years. The age-group of that community called *otu-ole* is given the responsibility to produce the ram on behalf of the community. However, before embarking on this task, they would be given a piece of white cloth, a native chalk, and an eagle's feather. All these are taken from the shrine in order to make the people become invisible as they work to catch the ram for sacrifice. During the ceremony, the *Oyiwa* buys a carton of beer, a crate of soft drinks, a bottle of schnapps, and a jar of palm wine. While the community may contribute the bottle of schnapps, it was nevertheless clear that they participate mainly to be feasted. The responsibility for entertaining the participants lies solely with the *Oyiwa*. For this general worship and celebration, all the chiefs appear in their chieftaincy regalia and gather around the shrine while the worship is going on. The attire worn by the *Oyiwa* is quite different from any other person's attire. He wears a white robe and a hat with an eagle's feather.

According to one of the interviewees, who is an *Oyiwa*, the ram brought for sacrifice is not killed. Rather, in the presence of all the worshippers, the chief priest will present the ram before *Nze,* makes incantations on it and offer it to *Nze* by saying: "*Kene bu ife/ebunu anyi wese-ni, as wa- nau ne ine-anyi*" (This is what we have brought to you this year). The assembly waits until the ram on its own accord stands up on its legs, enters the shrine, and walks to the backyard. With this, it is certified that the god has accepted the offerings and worship. Chief Patrick Enuademu recounted an instant in 2003 where the god nearly rejected the sacrifice. According to him the ram refused to stand up and would not walkthrough the shrine to the backyard. To avert this atrocity, the priests made series of incantations and plea for forgiveness of any offence the community might have committed. Eventually, their plea was heard as the ram stood up and walked through the shrine to the backyard. There are several prohibitions associated with *Nze*. For instance, it forbids Emu people from observing a ram slayed. To be watch the slaughter of a ram will cause the Emu person to become mad. The malady is curable with a body cleansing ritual. However, when the ram is killed, one can eat it. The same body cleansing ritual, when performed before Nze is able to cure any madness or psychological problems. This particular aspect of *Nze* belief, worship and sacrifice are still observed in Emu.

Nze forbids Emu people from having sexual relationship with a slave girl or an *osu* (outcast). A violation of this injunction attracts death. However, if a person who thus sinned in ignorance is afflicted with certain form of sickness that indicates infraction of *Nze* taboo. In such cases, the oracles is consulted and the victim is made aware of cause of the sickness. A ritual cleansing must be performed to restore such a person to good health. To perform this ritual the person is required to bring a white cock. The body of person is rubbed with the chicken and it is them thrown into the shrine. If the person commits this *alu* (sin) again, the person will have to repeat the cleansing process at the shrine. However, strict adherence to the ritual procedures has suffered certain setbacks. Emu indigenes resident in the cities visit the village for ritual purposes at their convenience. Also, Nze is only one of the many options available to them in time of problems. There could go to hospitals, seek Christian healing and consult other healers outside of Emu.

6.3 The Oyiwa

The *Oyiwa* is the chief priest of *Nze* and he has many taboos that he is to keep. It is forbidden for a menstruating woman to enter into his house and he is prohibited from even seating on a chair on which a menstruating woman had sat. In keeping to this injunction, the *Oyiwa* goes out with a leather skin and each time he enters a house, he spreads it on the chair before sitting down. He does this, because it is possible that a woman in her menstrual period may have sat on it. The *Oyiwa* maintains more than one house, such that when his wife begins her menstruation, she would move into the second house. The menstruating wife is not expected to come around the *Oyiwa's* main house nor allowed to cook for him throughout the period. The *Oyiwa* is also prohibited from eating "garri" (cassava flour) but not grain/corn meal. Whenever the *Oyiwa* is going to the shrine, he is not permitted to make any house calls. Finally, it is only the *Oyiwa* that sweeps the shrine. This practice has continued unchanged till the present time. Below is a typical prayer of the *Oyiwa* in his shrine:

> *Nze ne meye-o. Ni imeye ni egwe eeh, ni imeye ni egwe. Mbene, ni ke nde imeweye ni. Mbene, ni ke, nde inidi be merne. Nne ye yi nzu nkem, ne kene yi ni ne che umu m na mme. Nzu keni bu ke osa. Biko, deme osa anyi no obodo-ne, ne aka ife ojo. Onwê ru oria ojo di kita e. Biko, we fu ya na aru onye nyc na bata na obodo a. Biko we se ne yi ife oma. Anyi n'acho ife oma. Anyi n'acho ife oma. Anyi n'aclio ife oma, obu ife ojo. Biko osa ornu yi no iii uzo anya, ya man we. Ne ku me we anya. Kene bu oji n we se ni kita e. Ife m maru bu ke rnrnalu me ni, fodu ife nde mmuo me ni. Nji oji ne kene yi, na rio yi ni ke bia ko ni. Me me crc I no ne me me. Ke nti anyi nu ozi orna. Were oji, I bido na aru oru. Ya ni ke me oo! Ise*! (*Nze* do more that what you have done. Yes, you have tried much. Thank you for the ones you have done and the ones you are yet to do. This *nzu* is my personal offering in

> appreciation for protecting my children and me. This one I am offering to you is on behalf of all the Emu community. Please, protect every member of this community from all types of misfortune. There is a particular sickness that is grave AIDS. Please take it away from every woman coming into this community. Please bring good tidings for us. We are looking for good things for us. We are looking for good tidings for us. We are looking for good things and not bad ones. Please, protect all your children in diaspora, you know them. This is the kolanut brought before you today. I can only comprehend what humans do, not what the gods do. I am using this kola-nut to thank you and beg you for the one coming in future. Perform as you have been doing. Let our ears always hear good news, please. Take your kolanut, so that when you start working, you will go all the way!

While the taboos and observances are largely in place unaltered, there has been some changes to the worship of *Nze*. For instance, in the past, *Nze* worshippers abducted and killed people, using them as sacrifice. The bodies of such victims were kept in a place known as *Mgbugbu Onyenwoko* for three months, after which parts of the victims' bodies were brought as sacrifice to *Nze*. This practice is no longer observed. Those that were abducted and used for sacrifice were often murderers or slave hunters. Today in Emu, no one thinks of killing anyone as sacrifice to *Nze*. However according to an informant, during the war between Ogume and Emu, Ogume casualties were offered by Emu people as sacrifice to *Nze*.

Traditionally, *Nze* primarily protects Emu indigenes wherever they may be, recently, his protection has been extended to non-indigenes that are domiciled in Emu. As such any devotee or client may obtain *nzu* from *Nze* shrine in order to be made invisible when pursuing an ignoble act. However, *Nze* has now adopted new strategies to frustrate such people by making them vulnerable to their victims (Enuadernu, 2003). *Nze* also runs a program of assistance to his devotees, like helping them overcome humanly induced obstacles to a successful completion of whatever project or ambition they are pursuing. The god, *Nze*, has added the role of *Igbe* cult to its ever expanding portfolio, in that it now protects its worshippers from bad dreams, evil spirits, and witches. All that the devotee needs to obtain *Nze*'s protection are one piece of native chalk (*nzu*) from the shrine, a piece of white cloth, a feather of an eagle. These are tied together and put on their door post (Enuademu, 2003).

However, *Nze's* new widening portfolio has its attendant negative consequences. For instance, my informant believes that the local drug traffickers also use the piece of native chalk *nzu*, from *Nze* shrine to protect their business. Enuademu also narrated the following story: recently there was a court case against a member of the community. The case would have landed the Emu person in jail, if due process was followed. However, *Nze* was there to protect the person. According to my informant, Uboko worked with the Nigerian Army, and had a court case with his employers. He tried to run away but was apprehended. In the night a white cloth appeared to him and asked him to leave that environment but he was afraid because of the armed guards on duty. The white cloth of *Nze* assured him of a safe passage. He then stood up and walked past the guards without anyone questioning him. Uboko's journey out of the barracks had three obstacles (3 gates). He easily surmounted the first two but was accosted at the third gate. But surprisingly the piece of white cloth acted as a veil between him and the guards. It is believed that this is the kind of thing *Nze* does for his children these days.

In the light of the above discussions, it would be spurious to conclude that changes have not occurred within the *Nze* institution against the assertion of Enuademu who stated, that modernization has never changed anything. More pertinent perhaps is the position of another informant, Johnny Enwemike, who believed that the advent of Christianity and modernization, *ab initio*, did not change the pattern of *Nze*. Johnny Enwemike posited that *Nze* is still worshipped today as it had been in the past, but the areas of impact or change are in the number of believers that patronise the deity. Finally, many traditional worshippers have drifted away to join the Christian faith, hence, the number of worshippers is not as large as it was in the past. There is an ongoing change both in form and scope with respect to *Nze*.

6.4 Change and Continuity in the Beliefs and Rituals Concerning *Ani*

The god *Ani* is represented by the iroko tree (*anagba*) that stands at the centre of the Emu. It is believed that the tree was planted by the founders of Emu. The *Ani* is an indication that Emu is the owner of the land hence it is called the god of the land. *Ani* was and is worshipped by all that seek his intervention in their affairs. Additinally, every farming season, the community buys a fowl and gives it to the *Okpala-Uku* from Ogbolum, who uses it to prepare yam meal called *ebubu*. With this preparation the land is cleansed, purified, and readied for seedling.

While the iroko tree carries symbolic meaning for the community, the people nevertheless separate the tree from the god *Ani*. In 1980 the main tree in the city center was cut down as the people learnt from the oracle that the witches and wizards have tied up the good fortunes of the community and hid them at the apex of the iroko tree. As a result, there were many misfortunes in the city. A decision was taken by the community to cut down the tree. Since the tree was chopped, it is believed that Emu has been experiencing goodness. The removal of the iroko tree does not mean that the community has ceased to worship *Ani*, the people still worships *Ani*. Also, the ritual for the cleansing of the land still remains as in the past. Johnny Enwemike asserted that even Christians come for such cleansing. The only notable change is in the number of adherents. Another change concerns the amount of money spent as part of the offering to *Ani*. Whereas cowries was used in the past, today, the Nigerian currency (Naira) is now offered to the god. Finally, the *Okpala-Uku*, the chief priest of *Ani* was the only one charged with performing the worship of *Ani*, but these days, he is able to delegate his duties to someone else. Such a delegated person must, however, come from his family.

6.5 Change and Continuity in the Beliefs and Rituals of *Ossai*

As stated earlier in chapter two, this deity has its origin in Isokoland. Its' main function is to ensure procreation. It is also a personal god and as such every family keeps a shrine for it within their compound. There is no one central *Ossai* owned by the entire community. Originally, its function was to protect children. When a woman gives birth to a child, a cock is sacrificed to *Ossai* in the family when the child is three months old. This is to protect the child from misfortune, illness, sudden death and generally against infant mortality. Though, it is a guardian god, *Ossai* also makes a bad person restless until such a person confesses all his\her atrocities. In the olden days of inter-regional trade that was conducted by foot, *Ossai* as the guardian and protector of Emu people would cause an Emu man to escape unhurt when attacked by armed robbers in another town. However, with transportation, security escort services and the police the people no longer value the god for these services. Consequently, its worship has waned. Furthermore, contributing to the decline in the number of the devotees, especially the family units that formed the core of *Ossai* worshippers, are western education, modernization and Christianity. Modernization brought its new ways of rearing and training children. Dispensaries and healthcare systems assure a better and more certain health protection for children. Child mortality rate has also been reduced through improved maternity services and immunization, thereby assuring the decline in the importance of *Ossai* for the people.

Another setback is the emergence of another god called *Elishi* that seems to be filling the vacuum created by the decline in interest for *Ossai*. This new god is growing in reputation among Emu people as the god of protection and training of children. This god has its origin in *Umu-Ukpene* quarters in Etevie Street of Emu. The priest of *Elishi* is the *Ogene* of Emu. The priesthood of this shrine is by inheritance; it transfers from father to son within the same lineage. During the reign of *Okpala Ogbodo* of Ikosa at about 1711, there was a dispute between the chief priests *Osanebi* over the ownership of *Elishi*. It was alleged that *Okpala Ogbodo* suggested and insisted that the *Elishi* be made a communal property. The Chief priest Osanebi and his family refused. Nevertheless, the community went ahead and prepared their *Elishi*. The people started worshipping the new *Elishi* believing that it gives children but to their disappointment, the community experienced barrenness in the land for three years. During that period, menstruating women had no respite. Their blood flow refused to cease. It was at this time that a man called Ashebeta from Aradhe community, who lived in Emu, offered sacrifices to the Community *Elishi* in the hope that his wife will become pregnant. But his problem persisted for four years. So he got annoyed and went back to the old *Elishi*, where he offered sacrifices. It was then that his wife became pregnant and gave birth to a child. Thereafter the community abandoned their newly created *Elishi* and went back to the original *Elishi*. They pleaded with the priest, requesting that the old *Elishi* be made to serve as the communal deity instead of a private deity. Osanebi consented to this.

Just as Robert Baum observed while writing on the Esulalu people this new shrine did not completely replace the old one (Baum, 1999: 118).

The establishment of the new *Elishi* by the community therefore, did not erase the existence of the old *Elishi*. According to my informant, there are currently no fixed periods for offering sacrifices to *Elishi*. As long as the *Ogene* is ready, sacrifices sacrifice to *Elishi* can always be arranged. In appeasing *Elishi*, the *Ogene* now calls the name of the person on whose behalf the sacrifice is being offered and presents the request of the person. Dances to *Elishi* are however performed periodically because they occur in conjunction with the *Ukwuata* festival. The songs for this dance are not originally *Elishi* songs but *Ukwuata* songs, and they are only displayed during the *Ukwuata* festival. The belief is that barren women who participate in the worship of *Elishi* will become mothers. Although *Elishi* gives children to women, only the male worshippers are allowed to see the *Elishi*. Any woman that sees the *Elishi* will have to offer sacrifices to *Elishi* to appease it. Such woman will be required to buy a bunch of plantain, ten tubers of yam, a ram, and pepper. *Elishi* forbids the eating of any cassava product by its priest. A menstruating woman does not greet the *Ogene*. If by mistake such a woman greets the *Ogene*, he will not answer. If he responds to her greeting, the woman's menstrual flow will cease. The woman will have to bring one chicken to the *Ogene* for cleansing. The *Ogene* is not allowed to sleep under the same roof with a woman during her menstrual period. The god *Elishi* will not be effective if the *Ogene* violates any of it rules and regulations.

The shrine of *Elishi* is still in existence today, but with Christianity and Western education, women no longer offer sacrifices to *Elishi*. Enwemike, an informer, observed that Christianity has really eaten deep into the fabrics of Emu traditions and has destroyed its values. The traditional priests now charge Christians higher than normal price when they come to the shrine (Enwemike, 2003). In the olden days, a separate hut was built where a woman resides during her menstrual period. But with colonialism and its attendant changes, a woman now sleeps on the same bed with the husband during her menstrual period and even 'crosses legs' with him. It is believed that, these changes are responsible for the decline in the value of *Elishi*. In spite of these ongoing changes, adherents of *Elishi* still firmly assert that any barren woman will conceive the very moment she offers sacrifices to *Elishi*. They also lay claim that *Elishi* is able to cure fibroids in women. For cure, an afflicted woman is made to drink water from *Elishi*.

No one knows the content of this water. The efficacy of the water is presumed to lie in the *Ogene* who speaks to the shrine, chants, and performs the necessary sacrifices.

6.6 Change and Continuity in the Rituals of *Ikenge*

Ikenge came to Emu through the founder of the Community who gave specifications on how to observe and serve it. *Ikenge* is the god of success. Associated with it is a religious festival that was described in chapter two. *Ikenge* festival is held at the end of the farming season, following the *Ukwuata* festival. It is an opportunity for the citizens to celebrate the success that they have recorded through the farming season.

Everyone has an individual *Ikenge* which could be symbolised by a cutlass or a carved wood. There is no specific time for its worship of personal *Ikenge*. Anytime the individual is happy with his *Ikenge*, probably because of his successes, he can offer sacrifices to his *Ikenge*. However, the offering of sacrifices to individual *Ikenge* depends on when the community's *Ikenge* festival takes place. The festival usually lasts for a period of nine days starting from an Eke market day. During the communal festival, no one is expected to fight or quarrel. During the celebration, all the clan chiefs come together at the *Onotu-Ukwu*'s palace to make a goat offering to *Ikenge*. On the market day following the sacrifice, individuals celebrate their successes publicly and by proclaiming the successes achieved during the past year. Someone that has made lots of money for instance will say: "*Ikenge ye nu m ego e. Obulu shi Ikenge e ye nu m aka. a ma lum ele no ka di nu m. Osa ife nwe ni. Ikenge ye nu m*" (*Ikenge* gave me this money. It would have been the other way if *Ikenge* had not helped me. All the things I have now, *Ikenge* gave them to me).

However, people no longer publicly attribute their successes to *Ikenge*. In the words of Enyabegwu,

> People no longer say, 'Ikenge provided them whatever they achieved'. It is the Christian God' these days, so that nobody will say one is worshipping juju (Enyabegwu 2003).

The ninth day of the communal celebration is a day of dancing and joyous celebration. The family eats and drinks together. Generally, if there are any serious issues to be discussed among the members of the family, this is the day for that such discussion take place. If a man had a medicinal herb that he has been hiding from his children, he will at this period reveal it to the children.

The celebration of *Ikenge* has changed a lot from what it used to be in the past. In the words of Ikusarna Abanum, this change can be attributed to Christianity. This is because in Christianity involves the fellowship of converts where they obtain sermons and teachings. According to Abanum, the Christian teachings make believers meek and forgiving. He regrets that traditional religion adherents have no form of assembly where they could discuss the 'good' values of their profession. In conclusion, the interviewee state that, when people saw the benefits of a Christian God, they started drifting to Christianity. Furthermore, many Emu people now live outside the Emu community, as a result, many are unable to attend the annual festival.

Part of the *Ikenge* festival is the *Inwu-Igbu* ceremony that is exclusively observed by those who have killed people. The significant feature of this aspect of the *Ikenge* festival is the presence of the *Okuma*. According to an unpublished work titled "Emu Kingdom", by the Heritage, History and Culture Committee of the Emu People, *Okuma* is a ritual war drum. It is carved out of a big tree trunk and covered at one end with human skin. Anyone who has never killed a human being cannot step on the *Okuma*. On the day of the ceremony, participants will climb the *Okuma* to celebrate and symbolize how they over powered their enemies and killed their victims. Anyone who killed a person and did not participate will be caused psychologically disturbed by *Okuma* and eventually will be made mad. This belief owes the view that the spirt of a human being is different from that of an animal. Human spirits according to the interviewee cause spiritual disturbance in the life of the person who has killed another human being. It is important to state that an Emu does not kill another Emu person. One may kill a stranger in self-defense or anyone disturbing the peace of the Community. However, if an Emu accidentally kills another, such a person cannot participate in the *Okuma* dance. This is because his actions will be analogous to "harvesting unripe palm fruits".

lgbudu is another event that often comes up during the *Ikenge* festival; however it is strictly speaking not an integral part of the *Ikenge* festival. It is a service of songs\burial performed for deceased members of the *Ogbu* society. The *Igbudu* was observed in honor of those warriors who had killed another human being during their lifetime. At the death of such a person, a mat is woven into the shape of a coffin; this they call *Igbudu*. The *lgbudu* ceremony is different from the *Ibe-Okpa* ceremony. According to the unpublished work "Emu Kingdom", *Ibe-Okpa* entails the severance of a cock in the midair, in front of a mock casket of the deceased. Thereafter, the *Okuma* drum is left in front of the casket for seven consecutive days in honour of the dead heroes. There is an *Igbudu* for every dead person, however, the Igbudu is specifically in honor of a person who was able to kill another person. Thus, this is a historical practice. For such a person, a goat is sacrificed for the *Igbudu* and a cock is also brought for the sacrifice. The cock will be beheaded with one stroke of the cutlass. The lifeless body of the cock is then held before the mock coffin (*Igbudu*) while the performers chant and *Igbudu* members hold their cutlasses in salutation around the *Igbudu*. Then they hit their cutlasses on the *Igbudu* saying, "*Je se Ic enwe yi ne aka Akpu-Ukwu, We je bido ije*" (Go and clear yourself from Akpu-Ukwu before you embark on this journey). After this ceremony the *Okuma* is kept in the dead man's place for nine days. At the end of the nine days, another cock is sacrificed to *Okuma* before it is returned to the house of the head of *Igbudu*. The head of this group is called "*Odede-Igbu*"; the position is acquired on the basis of seniority.

During the *Ikenga* festival, young men wear their skirt-like regalia, carry their masquerades (*Ochu*) and perform for the community with their cutlasses in their hands. The highlight of this masquerade dance is when the *Ochu* dancers are challenged to a cutlass-duel in order to test the efficacy of their charms. If the challenger is not "strong", his cutlass will fall off his hand and the *Ochu* will laugh at his folly. However, there have been instances where some *Ochus* have been suffered machete cuts. According to an informant, in such situations, the cutlass that was used must have been laced with "medicine" more powerful than the charm of the *Ochu*. However, where the *Ochus* possess superior medicines, they invariably defeat their challenger.

There is an ultimate type of medicine called "*Elekali*" that can be used during the duel. *Elekali* literally means, "no other power is superior". It practically defies the power of *Mbubu*. For Enuademu (2003) Christianity has not in any way diminished the power of *Elekali* in the community because increasing number of young men are embracing it, especially for protection against gunshots. This use of *Elekali* by young men is a recent development. It started when guns began to be used in the prosecution of wars. An example is the aforementioned *Emu-Ogume* conflict of 1995.

The process of religious change as shown in above instances is not cumulative, yet unmistakable and systematic when viewed in a wider regional and historical perspective. The *Ikenge* festival, *Okuma*, *Igbudu,* and *Ochu* have all experiencing ongoing changes. This is not to say that there has not been evidence of continuity to aspects of these practices. Between the polar ends of change and continuity are middle positions, which will include, according to Kalu (1978: 15):

> Continuities at point of contact or correlations; trans-valuation of native symbols where traditional symbols are acquiring new meaning; substitution, where new faith absorbs ingredients of the traditional as a survival or acculturation process; and transformation, where completely new symbols and values are created in the confrontation of the old and the new.

In the past, a warrior who was able to subdue and kill an enemy would climb the *Okuma* to proudly announce to the community that he killed another human-being. However, the informer, Enuadernu, lamented that this is no longer the case. Those that kill these days do not disclose themselves for fear of prosecution. Supporting him, Eyabegwu noted that, due to the modernisation, people no longer rejoice or pronounce that they have killed somebody. For instance, if someone puts an eagle feather on his head, which signifies that he had killed another human being, he would be accosted on the road and asked what the feather means. Most likely the person questioning him might be a law enforcement agent. That is why *Igbudu* is no longer what it used to be. However, another informer noted that:

> It is not correct to say that the advent of modernisation has been a deterrent to the celebration of *Ikenge* by the members of the *Igbu* society. They still come out to observe the festival. We cannot celebrate *Ikenge* without the members of the *Igbu* otherwise it will no longer be *Ikenge* festival.

Still vexed by the general belief that things have changed due to influence of modernisation, Enuademu strongly expressed his belief in the following words:

> It is wrong to say that *Igbu* is no longer what it used to be because of the uncommonness of wars among tribes these days, otherwise, *Ikenge* should have been a

> thing of the past. It is absolutely wrong to think that one would just be pushed to kill because he wants to prove that he is a member of the *Igbu* society. An Emu man, who lives as far away as the western states of Nigeria may be attacked by enemies and in self-defense may kill the attackers. He would definitely come home to see the head of *Igbu* (*Ododo Igbu*) and announce to him the feat he achieved far away from home. So it is not that our people look for trouble or who to kill.

To Enuademu Christianity and the establishment of Police Stations have not stopped the observance of the *Ikenge* festival. It is still how it used to be.

6.7 Change and Continuity in the Beliefs and Rituals Concerning *Igba*

Igba is the deity that is believed by the Emu people to protect its worshippers from gunshots and cutlass wounds. This deity has no definite origin, but legend has it that the entire community at one time decided that they wanted it. In the olden days, children were abducted from the community and killed. The people were in constant fear of the persistent attacks from neighboring communities. Therefore the community invited a man to prepare a shrine for it. The first shrine was located at the Ikosa quarters of the community and the next was the Ebilije quarters. These two *Igba* shrines were very effective and active. Because the man did a very good job, he was taken to Emu-Obiogo, the next community in the clan where he built another shrine and from there, he was taken to Emu-Obodoeti among others. At Emu-Ebendo where the man did the final preparation, the people decided not to allow the man to go back to his village, because, it would be possible for the man to withdraw the power that determines the effectiveness of the *igba*. They slayed him and sacrificed his blood to *Igba* thus assuring the effectiveness of the *igba* cult in Emu community up till the present. It is believed that if one takes a ring and drops it in the pot water in the shrine and then wears it on his arm, the person will become immune to gunshots and machete cuts. Nobody can become the chief priest of *igba* without the consultation of the oracles. The oracles reveal to the *Okpala-Ukwu*, who in turn, reveals it to the person that he has been chosen for such responsibilities.

All the various shrines in the five clans of Emu have the same prohibitions. On the day that *Igba* is worshipped everyone contributes money to buy a fowl and a dog. These are used as sacrificial animals. Then a town-crier is sent to announce the day that *Igba* would be worshipped so that every dog owner will tie elephant grass round the neck of their dog. Also, no fowl is allowed to roam about else such stray animals are killed and taken to the *Igba* shrine. The dogs are free to roam about but they must have the elephant grass around their necks, lest they are killed and taken to the *Igba* shrine for sacrifice. The worship of *Igba* prohibits the consumption of snails and fused plantains. Another significant prohibition of *Igba* is that anybody who had entered the *Igba* shrine is forbidden from seeing a baby that is less than nine days old. If this is violated, the child will die.

There is a major drift from how *Igba* was worshipped in the past to how it is worshipped today. In the past, any sacrifice is offered only in the presence of the whole community, however, this is no longer the case. Anyone with money can engage the chief to perform the rituals according to the taste of the paying client. This private ceremony is to stop others from sharing in the proceeds of the sacrifice. The belief among devotees however is that *Igba* still lives up to the expectations of the people.

6.8 Change and Continuity in the *Ukwuata* Festival

The *Ukwuata* festival was and still celebrated so that Emu people can appease their ancestors (*Nde Iche*). At the end of the farming season, the *Ukwuata* festival which is the New Yam festival is celebrated. This festival is found common to Ukwuani speaking people. Once it is time for *Ukwuata* festival, the *Okpala* conveys a meeting of the two quarters that make up the community and a date is fixed for the celebration. On the chosen date, every young man, including the local vigilante group, will go to hunt. Young men will camp for nine days in the bush where the *Ukwuata* shrine is situated. During this period any animal that is killed or fish that is caught is brought to the camping place called *Uno Ukwuata* (house of *Ukwuata*). Only animals killed or fish caught during this general hunting is brought to the *Ukwuata* house. The animals and fish are to be cooked there and offered as a sacrifice in the *Ukwuata* structure.

At the end of the nine days, the camp is dismantled and for another nine days, people will remain at the camp site. On the fourth day of the second 9 days, the *Ukwuata* will be met by a group of dancers from the two quarters of the community. The two groups of dancers then proceed to the palaces of the two *Okpalas* to dance for them. Today, in place of these traditional dancers, different social and traditional clubs now perform. The *Ukwuata* festival is brought to an end by an act known as *Ichu-Ifeu,* (meaning "cleansing of the land and extermination of evil things".

The *Ichu-Ifeu* is conducted by the women, all holding burning lamps (woods) in their hands. At dawn, these women walk throughout the streets with their burning lights with which they exterminate the evil spirit in the town. The other group of people involved in this process is the age group known as *Otu-Onuogbe.* This exercise is considered necessary because, it is believed that in the course of the celebration of *Ukwuata* festival, many evil spirits are present in the whole town. *Ichu-Ifeu* is, therefore, done to tell these evil spirits that the festival is over and that they should go back to their various destinations.

Following the *Ukwuata* dance is the performance of the masquerade *Olu* comes. This masquerade makes two other appearances, the last appearance is on the *Orie* day. On this last day, the *Ichu-Ifeu* is conducted to mark the end of the *Ukwuata* festival. The performance by the masquerade is still in existence although it has not performed for some time now. This is because, the person that beats the *Ukwuata* is no longer alive and there has not been a replacement for him. There is no particular age-grade that is responsible for dancing the *Olu.* In the past, anyone who knows the dance-steps is selected to join in the *Olu* dance. But presently, the age grade known as *Otu-Onuogbe* that is found in each quarter of the town is charged with producing a dancer to represent their street.

The most significant aspect of the *Ukwuata* festival is the dance itself, but it has suffered some alterations in the recent years. Each year, the family that should produce the *Ukwuata* dancer consults the oracle to nominate the dancer for that year from among the members of that particular family. The family then offers sacrifices to appease the god to ensure the safety and good health of the dancer. For this dance, the chosen dancer must be fortified spiritually. Therefore, certain sacrifices are made to the gods, for it is not an ordinary feat to perform the dance steps. The dancer therefore must be "bathe" spiritually. Narrating his own personal experience, the informer, Enyabegwu said he had to cure himself for three years after dancing *Ukwuata.* "In the past it was like war, but these days it is no longer that way. The high level of wickedness of the past does not exist anymore", he said.

The *Ukwuata* Masquerade which the dancer carries on his head is made of carved wood. Originally, the carving was adorned with a life white eagle, but these days, it has become extremely difficult to get such an eagle. This could be attributed to the speedy deforestation of the communities in the light of modernization. Enyabegwu confirmed that, they used to go to the *okpokolo* forest, which was on the border of Emu or they would go to the forest in Ebo town to catch the eagle. In the absence of an eagle, a monkey is now used. The monkey is tied to the *Ukwuata* and covered with a piece of white cloth. The interviewee maintained that these days, it is increasingly still difficult to also get a monkey because of severe hunting. So most times, the people are left with the option of just using a piece of white cloth. This same piece of white cloth is used year after year and is left in the custody of the last dancer, who then passes it on to a current dancer. In the past, the *Isue* (hunters) provided the community with the creatures needed for this dance, these days however, they are purchased in the market.

After the *Ukwuata* dance, if the eagle is still alive, it is kept so that other communities that are yet to celebrate their *Ukwuata* could use it. On the other hand, if the eagle dies during the performance, the *Ukwuata* dancer could elect to eat it. It will not be out of place to say that the *Ukwuata* of these days has been polished. The camping that was done by all the young men in the past is now done by the *Otu-Ole*. The various ingredients that gave the festival its uniqueness have are rarely obtainable. The role of hunters has disappeared as young men no longer find hunting a viable vocation. Moreover, in the past, there used to be benefits that accrued to persons that accept to dance the *Ukwuata*. The age-grade responsible for producing the Ukwuata dance, as earlier stated, was the *Otu-Ole*. Today, the person whose turn it is to dance *Ukwuata* may get another to dance on his behalf, if he does not want to do the dance himself. Previously, the dancer was entitled, as a form of reward, to harvest palm nuts freely for five years. But today, there are people who are envious of such great reward given to the young man. Often times this displeasure drives them to poison the young dancer. This is why people who are not "strong spiritually" do not allow their sons to participate in this dance. In fact, very few young men are interested in the dance today.

6.9 Change and Continuity in the *Iwaji* Festival

At the end of each farming season, Emu people celebrate *Iwaji* festival. With this feast, the people are officially permitted to eat the newly harvested yams. It is also a time to make sacrifice to, and honor the yam god, *Ifejioku*. It is important to note that because the festival has not been observed in a few years does not mean that an individual cannot go to his farm to harvest his yams neither is an individual deterred from eating his new yams. There is however, a group of people who are prohibited from eating the new yams unless the festival is observed. These are those performing the rituals for becoming medicine men (*dibie*). If they eat the new yam before the festival, they will be spiritually attacked by the gods. When such an attack occurs, the person will require some cleansing.

At the end of the farming season, all the chiefs assemble in the palace of the *Okpala-Ukwu* and fix a date for the celebration of *Iwaji* festival. The festival last nine days. On the ninth day, all the quarters in the community contribute together twenty tubers of yam to the *Okpala-Ukwu* from the Ebilije quarters of the community. The Ogbonodi Street donates two big baskets (*abo*) of yam and the *Okpala-Ukwu* a basket of fish and a basket of different animal heads. Part of this collection is used to prepare the food consumed at festival and the rest is shared out to the different streets. Other ingredients needed for preparing the food for the feast are provided by the *Ada*, the eldest woman in the community. These ingredients include salt, pepper, potash, oil, etc. The food prepared during the festival is called *Otite*. *Otite* is a herbal vegetable collected specifically for cooking the soup used in eating the yam, which is roasted. The *Ada,* at the end of the feast, is given some yams, fish and meat.

This feast occurs only once a year after which individuals are free to serve their ancestors on their own. According to the Enyabegwu (2003):

> This feast is done with a view to seeking guidance from a person late parent. But the Christians say we are serving the devil. Who is the devil? My mother? My mother cannot be a devil. It is their mother that is a devil.

The most important part of the festival is the wrestling match that holds the ninth day of the festivity. On that ninth day, everyone in the community troops to the village square, where able bodied young men wrestle one other. Any reputable man that has a strong son prepares him for the match with medicine and herbs to assure his victory. These days, no one takes the wrestling matches seriously any more. No one cares if his son is defeated or not. This is because there has emerged other parameters for measuring superiority and earning prestige among the people. So, one does not find families preparing their sons for these matches as was practised in the past. Presently, more people are subscribing to the Christian faith and they are paying little or no attention to *Iwaji*. In the good old days, recalled Enyabegwu (2003)

> If a man takes a woman from your family unlawfully, the wrestling match was an avenue of carrying out a revenge. This was done by ensuring that you throw defeat everybody from that family, in order to disgrace its men. These days, nobody is interested in this, because people no longer appreciate or recognise the value of reputation and integrity achieved from such matches.

6.10 Continuity and Change in the Social Values of Emu People

Religious change has laid its weight on Emu people's social values, especially as pertaining to prohibitions or abominations. These prohibitions are twofold: those that are related to the desecration of the land and those that are morally and socially based. Some of these have been discussed earlier in chapter two. The value system and prohibitions of the Emu people is vast and require another book. However, one of the values that has experienced significant changes over time is discussed below.

6.11 Changes and Continuity in Emu Burial Rites

In the time past, when a matured, married man who is a chief dies, he was wrapped in a mat and carried into the evil forest; these days however, they are buried inside their compounds. After the deceased had been committed to earth, the family fire a canon twice to indicate that nobody should go to the farm the next day because it is considered a sacred day. The following morning, two canon-shots are fired again to confirm that the day is sacred. The last canon-hot is made to call the age-grade to come to offer their respect. This practice by the *Otu-Ole* age grade is a recent development, for in the past they did not come out after the last gun shot. When the corpse had been buried, a mat and leaf stalk from the palm tree is used to make the coffin for the dead man. However, today, this is irrelevant, if the deceased is buried at home or in the forest, a casket is used.

If the deceased is buried at home, the *Otu-Ole* age grade goes into the evil forest and calls his name, since it is believed that the decease joins his colleagues in the spiritual world the very moment he is buried. But if the corpse had not been buried, then there is no need to make the coffin for it. When the coffin has been made, a bunch of leaves was briefly scotched and placed to the coffin to symbolize the entrance of the spirit of the deceased into the coffin. The coffin is the covered with a white cloth. Yams are roasted in front of the coffin. If the deceased was a woman, water yam is roasted, and yellow yams, if it was a man. A kid is slaughtered and its blood sprinkled round the borders of the white cloth that covers the coffin.

Before the coffin is buried, women dance around the coffin; they dance to a special burial dirge. The food that is cooked for the dead person is meant to be consumed by the living. The ingredients for this food include; fresh calabash seeds, the head of an electric fish and yams. The soup is also intended for the deceased alone, as such it is not tasted by anyone. By not eating the food, the people confirm that they have no relationship with death. The food is prepared as sustenance for the dead to ensure that the dead does not starve in the new abode. As the coffin is lowered into the grave, water is sprinkled on it, this water is for the dead to drink after eating the food.

Following the internment, a burial ceremony is organized. On the fourth day of this gathering, a ritual is performed to completely separate the dead from the living. If the dead was a man, his wife provides the required ingredients for this ritual. Any matured goat found or seen roaming around is killed, whether it belonged to the deceased family or not. This was the practice in the past and no one raised alarm over such action, for it was well understood as part of the burial rites of a deceased. Today, the kid used for this ceremony is bought from the market to avoid been labeled a thief and thus risk legal actions. The goat is slaughtered to appease the gods so that the deceased is not judged for any ambition that he might have nursed but did not fulfill before his demise.

When the husband of a woman dies, a rite of final separation is performed before the burial. The woman lies on the same bed with the corpse of her husband in a position contrary to her deceased spouse, i.e., her head is to his feet. This rite establishes that they will never again sleep together as husband and wife, not even in her dreams. However, with modernisation, many women are no longer made to pass through the ordeal of sleeping with their dead husbands. While this practice is now negatively viewed, it is still a common practice, according to my informant, it is a taboo for a man's head to be touched by the feet of his wife. When that occurs, a sacrifice has to be offered to *Ani*.

As part of this rite, the woman was also asked to bring the last wrapper or cloth that her husband wore before his death and the one she too wore before his death. Both were included in the coffin. Three days after the death of a husband, the wife is taken at night by her family to the outskirt of the town, where her hair is shaved. This was to signify that the hair of the woman he saw and touched would no longer be there for him to see and touch and thus further cement their separation. It is interesting to note that these days enlightened women in the community no longer want to have their hair shaved as was done in the past.

Following the shaving rite, the woman washes her head with the warm water and she puts on a new set of clothes. With this, she signifies a complete severance of the relationship between her and the dead husband. The woman then stays indoors for three moons, mourning. However, a man whose wife died stays indoors for only nine days. My informant quickly pointed out that this must not be viewed as cheating on the part of men. According to him, if a woman died, the husband had more responsibility to take care of their property at home and in the farm, in order to cater for the children. There were some men that would not re-marry until a year after the death of the wife, because they considered this to the period of mourning. These days, many women are employed in various establishments. Thus it is increasingly difficult to keep women indoors for "three moons" to mourn their dead husbands. In these days of great individualism, women and men alike have to go to work in order to meet their responsibilities. Also, many families no longer offer the same assistance to women upon the death of her husband, as was done in the past.

As part of the burial rites, the first son of the bereaved woman did not eat from his mother, until she had gone and offered sacrifice to *Olor*. This occurs after the burial ceremony. If the son violates this prohibition, he will die, though not instantly. Thus, the family has the chance to offer sacrifices to the gods to save the son's life. Now, this aspect of the burial rites of the Emu people is almost completely eradicated as they are largely viewed as fetishism. City life, influence of other cultures and Christianity have eroded the rites among the people.

A rite called *Ibe Okpa* is performed when a woman dies. This involves the roasting of a fowl and cooking of yam at the side of the town that faces the village or quarters of the deceased. For instance, if the woman was from Abbi, the children of the woman will bring a fowl to the women in the family of the deceased woman. They will go to the side of the town at the entrance to Abbi. There, they will roast the fowl and cook the yam. The food is eaten there and some portion are left there as well. During the burial ceremony of a woman, her husband shall only appease her *Ofo* but after then, he hands it over to the eldest woman in the family. It will then become the responsibility of that woman to offer annual sacrifices to the *ofo*. In a home with no women, a male in that family is charged with this responsibility. It is viewed as indecent by the people if a man offers this sacrifice when there is a female in the home. Such a man is regarded as greedy.

The burial rites in some aspects of contemporary Emu culture are a synthesis of tradition and modernity. From the traditional point of view what exists today as burial ceremony is sometimes a brazen show of materialism. There is now a lot of display of traditional dances with Christian musical bands playing alongside western music. There are also now Christian wake service along with the traditional one, an unholy wedlock that has produced chaos in the eyes of traditional religious adherents.

Chapter Seven: Continuity and Change in Emu Religious Belief and Ritual Practices

The delicate balance between tradition and modernity in Emu has resulted in a kind of cross cultural integration. This delicate balance contributes to the softening of the effects of the drastic changes to the religious beliefs and ritual practices of the people. Some of these changes and their effects are discussed in this chapter.

7.1 Continuity and Change in Emu Productive and Protective Medicine

Productive and protective medicines are medicinal preparations used in connection with diseases and sickness. They are believed to steer away evil forces. Protective rituals are performed out of the people's response to perceived danger or even psychological fear of life itself. Emu people have a morbid fear for the power of destructive medicines. Dangerous and destructive forces could be employed by unknown persons at the slightest provocation to wreak havoc in their homes, families, and even on unborn children. Besides the fear of evil medicine, the people believe that natural forces can manifest their powers sometimes to the people's detriment. Therefore, numerous protective medicines are needed to ward off these various sources of evil.

7.2 Medicine for Memory: *Ogwu Akonuche*

In the remote past *ogwu akonuche* medicine was employed by the priests and medicine men to aid them in memorising traditions, ritual incantations, and numerous medicinal prescriptions. The traditional dancers and musicians used it to commit to memory songs and difficult dance steps. However, today it is used by students to help them study. Urbanization and the drift to the cities have assisted in transporting *Ogwu Akonuche* to other places. People now employed it in various works of life where good memory is required.

Also, there have been some changes to the ingredients needed for this medicine. In addition to what has already been stated in chapter three, the number of *Nkolo* fish (tilapia) has increased from one to seven. In the place of *Nguta* leaves are forty-nine *Ukpa* leaves. There are also changes to its preparation. All these items are put together in a pot and cooked as a soup for seven days. Using the left hand, it is drank with a spoon three times a day until it is all gone. However, there has been continuity in the words that are recited and the beliefs in the efficacy of this medicine. But unlike in the time past, when the medicinal substance was licked and incisions are made to the head, the common practice now is to swallow the soup and mumble the words of incantation secretly.

7.3 Rain Medicine: *Ogwu Mmili*

There are two types of *Ogwu Mmili;* these are *ogwu ifemmili* and *ogwu Idommili. Ogwu Ifemmili*, the most widely used in the community is grouped under good or productive medicine. It is the act of preventing rainfall from disturbing such occasions as, festivals, burials, and other social activities in the community. There are different methods for doing this, but the interviewee, for reasons he would not disclose, chose to tell only one method. According to Enwemike (2003) while it is raining or drizzling, the rain-maker goes to a flowing stream river to talk with the god of rain. Immediately afterwards, there will be sunshine. Although this medicine is considered to be a 'good' medicine, he sounded a note of warning, that it could be dangerous if the rain-maker is not spiritually strong. For instance, there is a method of preparing this medicine that involves cooking. If it is already raining and the rain-maker wants to stop it through the cooking method, lightning and thunder may strike while he is cooking the medicine. If the rain maker is not "spiritually strong" he will abandon the process or die in the act.

Different from the above, the act of making rain to destroy or disrupt a ceremony is seen as a bad act. This is known as *Ogwu Idommili* and it is employed by the rain-maker to spoil the joy of the celebrant and his guests for whatever reason. When this is the case however, the rain maker is susceptible to more danger because he is inadvertently doing a wicked act.

According to the informant, Enwumike (2003), just like in the past there are no particular criteria for becoming a rain-maker. If a medicine man likes someone he can pass the knowledge to the person. Sometimes he may demand a fee for this transfer of knowledge. There are however prohibitions that must be observed by a rainmaker, these prohibitions are still observed today. The rainmaker for example is prohibited from drinking water, eating food prepared with oil, or sometimes he must not eat through-out the process. This last taboo depends largely on the type of *Ogwu Mmili* he is preparing. All these injunctions are still in place.

The act of making rain or holding back rain has not stopped in the community. Even enlightened and educated people in the community still seek out rainmakers whenever they have a ceremony. This medicine also has other uses in the Emu community. According to Enwemike (2003), "If a person plants tomatoes and they are dying due to lack of rain, he can make rain to prevent the crops from dying." He however, insightfully said that Christianity has affected and changed the reception and acceptability of this kind of ritual acts in recent times. He concludes with mixed feelings that, "some people have joined Christianity and therefore do not believe in it any more. But there are still those who have firm beliefs in rain making and so still seek the assistance of rain makers when need be."

7.4 Medicine for Belly Ache: *Ogwu Efo-Olinwa*

This type of medicine with its prescription and is to cure all forms of belly aches. From the recent fieldwork in the community, new revelations concerning this medicine were obtained. According to a *dibie*, George Dakwa, there is a stomach illness that disturbs a woman, it is called *Olinwa* i.e., fibroid. He said these days, it is difficult to treat or cure this sickness because women have sex with anybody they come in contact with. He asserted that having multiple partners makes the wombs of such women to become infested with all kinds of diseases and should they be struck by *Olinwa*, it becomes almost impossible to cure. The issue of multiple partners is due to modernization and liberalization both of which have found expression in the sexual behaviours of the contemporary Emu society.

In the past, a woman will experience cramps before they start their period and then the pain ceases. But now, the pains continue throughout the period. In the words of George Dakwa (2003), if it was in the past, such an ailment would be cured through the preparation of some medicinal herbs.

Unfortunately, these herbs no longer have any effect nor do they cure the illness because these women have spoilt their wombs. From Dakwa's account, we are able to understand two things. Firstly, there is continuity in Emu religious belief and ritual practices of *Ogwu Olinwa*. There are no dramatic changes in its prescription or ingredients. There is however, strong decline in the belief concerning its efficacy. This is inferred from Dakwa shifting the blame for its failure to the "way-wardness of women". It is however important to add that with medical science and surgery, women inflicted with fibroids find excellent cure with physicians.

7.5 Medicine for Premonition: *Ogwu Ashima*

It should be recalled that *ogwu ashima* gives its user intuitive signs that could be described as premonitions. It enables the user to make decisions regarding all spheres of their life. It also gives the user an idea of the future. The prescriptions and ingredients needed for the preparation of this medicine have been extensively described in chapter three. However, Iyama Oguise, who is a renowned medicine man in Emu informed me that the signs given to a user of *Ashima* are varied and are sometimes dependent on what the medicine is trying to warn the user about. For instance, in the case of a younger sister to the user, every sign that the user receives on the left side of the body is a good sign. But if is on the right side, then it is a bad sign. If it is a sign pertaining to a younger brother, the reverse is the case. He stated:

> If as we are sitting here, I feel something biting me on the back of my left shoulder, I would tell you where they are speaking good of me. This is because a woman is my immediate junior (younger sister).

The informant then suggested that this kind of medicine is not inherited but is obtained through a careful understanding of Emu culture. According to him, every man has signs but it is because we do not understand these signs that we go contrary. For instance, if one is travelling, his body will tell him either to take the trip or not. Every man has signs but unless one studies them, it will not make any sense to him. He said.

> If my left toe itches, I will know that I am about to see good money and it is so for everyone. If it is the right palm and person has a younger brother, he should also expect something good.

Oguise further stated that there is no event that happens without signs. For instance, the signs could either be used by God or the ancestors to warn of an impending danger. *Oguise* emphasized that there is a bird called *okiri* whose presence is symbolic. According to him, if the bird perches somewhere around the place one is and started to sing, a person of understanding will be able to discern the message that the bird is conveying. The knowledge to interpret the song of the bird is obtained from elders through socialization. *Ashima*, according to the informant, is not a god, thus it is not worshipped. Rather, it is a medicine that gives premonition. The signs differ depending on what the mediciner's preparation. For instance, a particular medicine man could always make the user see a chameleon as a warning of impending danger. It is not important whether one sees the chameleon in a cage for sale for instance. Oguise, rather speaking in parables, stated:

> If one has a medicine for winning cases in court, he will definitely make trouble so that he could go to court, because if he does not go to court, he would not know if the medicine is effective or not.

It is not out of place to say that the presence of Christianity in Emu community has caused a decline in the number of those that believe in and work with signs. However, it is not true to assert from this premise, according to *Iyama Oguise*, that the potency of *Ashima* is becoming unnoticeable. This is because it is still effective for those who believe in it.

There is yet another medicine that has been developed over the years comparable to *Ashima*. This medicine is known as *Elieli gba nwata oseleka*. That is, "A child will always withdraw his hands any time he touches an electric fish (*Elieli*)". This charm is still in existence, it works by sending a shock to the raised arm of an attacker who for instance wields a cutlass. If the cutlass touches the user of the medicine, the hand of the attacker will become paralysed. However, the user of this medicine is prohibited from eating electric fish (*Elieli*). If in ignorance he eats *elieli*, the person will become ill and will require cleansing.

The basic items needed for the preparation of this medicine include one electric fish, a tuber of yam (*iji-olu*), *adalikegu* (herbs). These ingredients are cooked and in the course of the cooking words of incantations are said to fortify the medicine. However, there is a big change in the general acceptance of this medicine today. People now view it with contempt. Stressing this point, *Oguise* gave an example:

> In the past people were paid to go and kill. They brought back human heads which were used to prepare a medicine that protects someone in the bush. But these days, no sane person is willing to take on this kind of assignment. This charm has lost its value.

7.6 Medicine for undefined Sickness and Sufferings: *Ogwu Emo Na Liali Ne Esu Mmalu*

This is a type of ritual medicine that is used in curing diseases and in protecting users from evil. Its prescription and the ingredients have been mentioned and discussed in chapter four. The informant, Okeleka maintains that there are no structural or fundamental changes to the ingredients and prescriptions for this medicine. However, one cannot rule out minor adjustments in the ritual procedures, such that relates to the *dibie*, his background, and how he acquired his skills. As the name of the medicine implies, it is used to cure a type of illness within the t he bloodstream. The medicine has other uses as well. For instance, if someone wants to fight a user of this medicine, the moment the attacker hits the user, rather than the person that was hit, the attacker will suffer the pain. The resultant sickness goes through the attacker's blood stream and veins due to its effect. Okeleka (2003) rates this medicine as bad, and advised against its use. The use of this medicine is not as rampant as it was in the olden days although some people in the Emu community still subscribe to it for self defence.

7.7 Medicine for Prevention of General Poisoning: *Aju Ogwu*

Aju Ogwu has a primary and secondary function. It cuts across protective and therapeutic medicine. There are three types of this medicine. The medicine is used as an antidote for poisoning. The restriction against *aju ogwu* is that it must not be brought into a home else it will lose its efficacy and cause the destruction of the properties in the house. If it is taken to the farm, it will cause the crops to wither. This kind of *Aju Ogwu* can however, be employed by a person who desires revenge, i.e., 'bad medicine'. The other type of *Aju Ogwu* is used to detect poison in any food offered to the user. In such cases, the medicine will cause the hand of the user to shake and thus not allow the food to get to the mouth. Should the user get the food to his\her mouth, the medicine will induce vomit. Due to its tripartite function and the associated side effects and prohibitions, it is not very attractive these days, although it is still widely used.

7.8 Medicine against Gun Shorts: *Igwu Egbe Ufie*

It should be recalled that this medicine is used to protect the user from gunshots. As the name implies gunshots directed to the user will miss its target. This medicine was developed following the introduction of the gun to warfare. Prior to this time, the medicine widely used for protection was the *Ogwu Mma* (medicine against machete cuts). The advent of *Ogwu egbe ufie* heralded the decline in the use of *Ogwu Mma* (medicine against machete cut). Unlike in the past when the people armed with this medicine could not be wounded in an attack, there is an increasing loss of faith in the ability of the medicine to protect the user. Enyabegwu (2003) stated that this medicine is no longer active, because of the introduction of injections, used in curing various diseases. These injections destroy most protective medicine in the body. So, it is necessary to drink frequently the medicine and make an incision on the body in order to maintain its efficacy. There is evidence of continuity pertaining to the ingredients for the medicine. The prescription has also remained the same, except that the user may have to drink the medicinal preparation more often than in the past.

7.9 Continuity and Change in Emu Destructive Medicine

Among the people of Emu, destructive medicines are those that have evil effects on humans and the society at large. These types of medicines were the focus of chapter four. In this section a few of this medicine are discussed to highlight changes and continuity to it.

7.9.1 *Ogwu Igba Mkpa*: Shooting of Poison

Igba Makpa is to send missiles to a person. It is considered a wicked act among the people of Emu and according to my interviewee, it should not be encouraged. In the past, if two men were fighting over a woman, they would go to the wrestling arena during the annual wrestling festival and duel. The loser feeling so disgraced often ends up seeking for ways to harm the other man, and could resorts to *Ogwu igba mkpa*. The moment these missiles are sent to a person, it would begin to work like AIDS, because it destroys the body system. There are different kinds of *Ogwu igba mkpa. Mkpannu* is one of them. This is prepared with salt. As soon as this type is injected into the body, the whole missile will melt like salt and permeate the body system. Then all the body immune system becomes weakened and if the antidote is not immediately administered, that person would die.

During the course of my interview, Enwemike (2003) recalled what happened to his father, saying:

> When my father wanted to marry my mother, my mother's father was not in favour of that union. As a result of this hatred, he sent *Ogwu igba mkpa* to my father, which burnt two of his fingers. But because his own father (my paternal grandfather) had the antidote, it was cured. If it happens these days, we will end up in the grave.

It is worthy of note that with Christianity and modernization this medicine is no longer common. However there now seems to be a resurgence of this medicine due to the recent political activities that have engulfed the community. The quest to win the Local Government Council elections has now led many to acquire this kind of medicine to be used against opponents. Probably, this explains why some politicians suddenly slump and faint at rallies. The only criteria for the application of *Ogwu igba mkpa* is that the victim must be within sight of the user. The commonest antidote for this medicine is to return the missiles "back to the sender." This antidote is freely prepared for people because it is not harmful unlike the *Ogwu igba mkpa*.

7.9.2 Ogwu Eti Ada: Hit and Fall

Another ritual medicine that is termed bad medicine is *Ogwu eti ada*, it is used for fighting. The medicine translates to "hit and fall". *Ogwu eti ada* was discussed in chapter three. From various interviews with Enuademu (2003), there are two other types of *Ogwu eti ada*-the male and female. According to him, the female type is not as strong as the male that can kill. When the male type is used the victim either dies instantly upon been hit or when he gets home after been hit. However, the striking difference between the *Ogwu eti ada* of chapter four and the one discussed here is in the ingredients. The ingredients needed to prepare the *Ogwu eti ada* are as follows; a ring, pumpkin seed, bark of palm tree struck by thunder, the heart of a toad, water from coconut fruit that fell prematurely from the tree, *kai-kia* (locally brewed gin).

The effect of *Ogwu eti ada* on the victim is that it causes the victim to fall to the ground. Unless the victim is kicked, he would not stand up. However, even if he stands up, after seven days, his hands and legs will become paralysed like the palm three struck by thunder. But this is not the case with the *ogu eti ada* of chapter Three where the victim is kicked on the head and he stands up. The victim become weak, confused and unable to speak, but eventually will regain health after receiving the antidote. The use and application of this medicine is now frowned at within the community. Anyone found using it is brought before the council of chiefs and is made to pay for the ritual cleansing and the cost for healing the victim.

7.9.3 *Ogwu Igbo Mmalu Onu*: Medicine to Cause Madness

This medicine was extensively discussed in chapter three. This medicine originally was used to make a victim insane. Today, it is used to place curse on people. Otherwise there have been no changes to this medicine. The medicine is still applied early in the morning as before. The user still faces the sun and spits out the ritual preparation. A person can place a curse on anybody including their children, by facing the sun and saying curse words. Whatever curses are spoken at that time will manifest in the lives of those so cursed. Enwemike stated that curse can however, be remedied. In his words:

> A woman that went stark naked to place a curse on her children will also go naked to withdraw the curse. She is required to say that she was angry when she cursed them. After this ritual, the effects of the curses will become nullified.

Enwemike emphasized that the root cause of curse is extreme anger; it is a common sight within the community to see someone cursing another, just because s\he is not happy with what the person has done. Most times they utter words like, "Let the person not see the light of day."

Enwemike however observed that the teachings of Christianity have helped to lessen these acts. *Ogwu ibo mmalu onu*, according to him, is no longer as effective as it used to be because the people now ignorantly eat what they were forbidden to eat. For instance, the eating of fused plantain. But these days, when one travels to the city and eats in the restaurants, he does not know whether the plantain that was served was fused or not. Also, the user should not walk under a rope used for hanging clothes to dry. But Enwemike laments that, "today all these prohibitions are not obeyed. So, the effects of the *Ogwu ibo mmalu onu* have been weakened by modern influence."

7.9.4 *Ogwu Iwa Ugboko*: Medicine of Command

The power of the *Ogwu Iwa ugboko* was displayed during the Emu-Abbi communal clash of 1981. This story as narrated by Enyabegwu (2003) will also show the efficacy of *Ogwu Ashima*, *Ogwu egbe ufie* and *ogwu elekeli gba nwata ose le aka*. During the war, Okolijenegu, the leader of the army from Abbi, who was reputed to be "strong" in his medicine - *Ufie*, approached Emu. As he was leading his army, there was drumming. Before he left Abbi, he took with him a small calabash (*Onunu*), which contained his *Ogwu iwa ugboko*. On his way, he chanted, "if there is anybody waiting for me on the road, the person or persons should go to the village square and wait for me there, because no man waits for me on the road." His chanting had immediate effect, Amudo from Emu responded and came out from where he was laying ambush and called others to come out. He told everyone to go back home because nobody was coming from Abbi for any war. Every Emu fighter came out from their various hide out wondering why they had not gone to their farm instead.

All this time, Ekpeti-Ukwu, the leader of the Emu warriors, was sitting at the centre of the road snorting tobacco. Meanwhile, Osoku, another warrior was reluctant to go because of the signs from *Ashima*. As the men of Emu were going back home, they got to a kolanut orchard and asked Ugoji, one of the fighters, to climb the kolanut tree and pluck some kolanuts for them to chew. When he climbed the tree he saw in a distance Okolejenegu and the host of the Abbi army coming for the war. Immediately, all the men from Emu dove back into the bush and left Ekpeti-ukwu, who sat in the centre of the road with his gun and tobacco box. Okolojenegu, from a distance, commanded Ekpeti-Ukwu to go back to the village square, because that is where he was going to fight. Ekpeti-Ukwu, in response, said to him that he will die a miserable death. He also told Okolojenegu that it was his last day on earth because of his decision to attack Emu.

Okolojenegu brought out his own chair and sat opposite Ekpeti-Ukwu, while two girls fanned him. He commanded that Ekpeti-Ukwu be shot dead. Several rounds of shots were fired at Ekpeti-Ukwu. However, because of his *Ogwu egbe ufie*, instead of bullets, smoke was coming out of the guns. After so many attempts, Ekpeti-Ukwu stood up and beckoned on the other Emu warriors in ambush to come out and there they engaged one another. At the end, most Abbi men died, but Okolojenegu and a few "strong" ones remained. The warriors from Emu turned on Okolojenegu, and started shooting at him, but nothing happened to him. Not a bullet touched him. At a point, nobody had bullets anymore. A special gun that was made with *Ogwu-Elekeli* was then shot at him and he fell down. His body began to decay and rot at the spot. And so the warrior died.

The highlight of the above story was the introduction of the *Ogwu-Elekeli*. Prior to the war in the story, there was no antidote for *Ogwu Egbe Ufie*. Also, *Ogwu Iwa Ugboko* has continued to be an enigma to the people. Unlike in the past when there were inter communal wars, the medicine is currently employed to recall family members that are in distant lands. Such victims of *Ogwu-Iwa Ogboko* return home without understanding why they came home.

Conclusion

Change is a permanent feature of a man's life and has always been an essential aspect of the cultural history of different African peoples. The case of Emu people provides a good illustration. E. A. Ayandele in an article review captioned "The Collapse of 'Pagandom' in Igboland" alluded to the demise of indigenous traditional religions by noting that:

> …the Christianisation of the Igboland was nothing short of an epic. Not even in Ijebuland, similarly physically conquered by the British invaders and where the gospel achieved an amazing success were the walls of 'Pagandom collapsed Jerichowise as in Igboland… (See Ejizu, 1989: 134–135).

Different from Ayandele whose assertion above does not really reflect the contemporary situation in Emu society, is Simon Ottenberg's (1959: 139) assertion that "the introduction of Christianity has provided people with religious options. Consequently, they are able to choose and many Igbo have accepted Christianity without rejecting completely their traditional religious beliefs". Similarly William Bascom and Melville Herskovits cautioned on the dangers of overt conclusion about the discontinuity of African religions due to Christianity. They remarked that:

> Despite the intensity of Christian missionary effort...which has marked the history of various parts of Africa, African religions continue to manifest vitality everywhere. This is to be seen in the worship of African deities, the homage to the ancestors, and the recourse to divination, medicine and other rituals (Bascom and Herskovits, 1959: 3).

Realignments and shifts in allegiance are found among Emu people due missionary proselytization that has aided a breakdown in aspects of traditional world-view. As has been described in a different chapter, Christian religious influence, neo-colonialism, a new economic system, urbanization, science and technology constitute external and internal factors of change in Emu. But despite these changes, there is continuity on the one hand and decline on the other, for instance, there is the prevalence of traditional priest-craft, but a decline in the use of traditional medicine and the concomitant belief that injections (e.g., inoculations) introduce substance into the body that weakens the efficacy of traditional Emu medicine. It was also observed that some of the people who changed to new religions, with the hope of greater socio-political benefits like Adame in Chapter Six, were ultimately disappointed. The resultant disillusion, be it with aspects of the new or of the old, has produced religious syncretism. In support of this observation, one of the informants narrated a story about how the Christians visit them (medicine men) to seek solutions to their problems. When this happens, they (the medicine men) will charge the Christians higher fees. The medicine men have continued to emphasize that regardless of the intermittent breaks and gaps in the religious beliefs and ritual practices, there are traditional medicines that have persisted; while some have declined others have acquired new port folios and functions. Akama aptly captured the situation by noting that:

> External trade and secular education also helped to open the minds of many Nigerians to new ideas and new horizons of human endeavours. Indeed, external trade and educational pursuit had shattered the microcosmic boundaries of the various originally enclosed Nigerian communities. Therefore, the exhibition of new orientation acquired by such members began to give tremendous influence on the traditional religion and culture (2001: 28).

As already described, the resilience and revival of the indigenous religion and culture caused the demise of the Catholic Church in its first phase of its existence in Emu-Unor. Some Christians in the community who claimed to be "true" believers turned out be pragmatists who saw nothing wrong in practicing "small" medicinal rituals alongside their Christian faith. They sought additional protective measures from good medicine like *Njo Puazu, Ogwu mma,* and *Ogwu Egbe* among others. Consequently, Messenger (1958: 292) showed that among the Anang Ibibio people:

> Missionaries have met their strongest resistance in trying to alter Anang beliefs in reincarnation, the power of oath spirit and the existence of 'witches', Ghost and evil medicine.

The daily stress of rural living, the political and economic uncertainties as well as the numerous "problems of life" make the use of 'good' medicine necessary. Following the rising demand for traditional medicine in certain areas, there has been a rise in the number of professional and lay medicine men. People adopt and adapt various types of rituals to deal with different circumstance. *Ogwu Akonuche*, the medicine to aid memory, which was originally used by medicine men and priest to aid the retention of rituals, religious traditions, incantations, and numerous medicinal formulas, is now commonly sought by students who believe that it will enhance their memory and they will learn better. *Ogwu egbe* and *Ogwu mma* medicine for protection against gunshot and cutlass cuts are now being by armed robbers and smugglers as well as by the members of the armed forces.

The tensed and charged atmospheres that traditionally accompanied the rituals and sacrifices have now given way to a casual attitude and relaxed atmosphere both on the part of the medicine men and their clients. It is not now common to see younger *Dibie* or diviners invoke the Christian God for additional power when they prepare traditional medicines. And when Christians come for consultation, objects of Christianity are often utilized.

Persons who are ill or injured often seek relief from both traditional medicine makers and medical doctors.

It is important to note that things such as the abrogation of traditional judicial system of justice, oath taking, trial by ordeal and traditional ways of detecting sorcerers by the Nigerian state has by default led to an increase in the belief and use of evil medicine. By sending some of this practice underground, they seem to acquire validity. Consequently, there is increase in the patronage of the *dibie* by the people seeking protective medicines. In all, it has been shown that in the transition from the traditional to the modern, made possible Christianity and colonialism, the belief in and practices of ritual medicine remain strong and current among the Emu people. In deed, "there is no African culture which has not been afflicted in some way by European contact and there is none which has given way to it" Bascom and Herskovits (1959: 3).

Despite the fact that medicinal rituals in Emu are at times successful and at other times not so successful, Emu people stick to their belief in the efficacy of such medicinal, especially sorcery. Following Pritchard (1976: 463), it may be because:

> They do not think very much of the matter. It is an accepted fact that the more potent medicines achieved their purposes. The best proof of this is experience, particularly the mystical evidence of oracular revelations.

The lack of futility and incongruity in the efficacy of ritual medicine as contained in the mindset of Emu people may be because they operate by faith rather than subjecting their actions to empirical verification. This tenacious grip to ritual medicine is best illustrated with Horton (1972: 25) assertion, that:

> Typically, a sick man goes to a diviner and is told that a certain spiritual agency is "worrying" him. The diviner points to certain of his past actions as having excited the spirit's anger and restore health remedial action, which will appease this anger and restore health. Should the client taken the recommended remedial action and yet see no improvement, he will be likely to conclude that the divine was either fraudulent or just incompetent, and seek out other expert...if after this the client should still see no improvement in his condition he will move on to get another diviner and so on.

It is thus clear that the people are pragmatic, they seek solutions regardless of its source. The Emu search for medicine is purpose driven. In this regard, it is hard to imagine that the Emu *dibie* is out to manipulate or indulge in trickery but to produce efficacious ritual medicines. Thus, the lack of empirical explanations for some Emu beliefs and ritual practices is not a sufficient basis to dismiss them. Of importance, is that the study of Emu worldview and medicinal ideas reveal their mindset and communicate their ideals as well as underscore their dynamics in the ever changing culture.

Bibliography

Published Books

Abimbola, W. (1975). *Sixteen Great Poems of Ife*. Geneva: Unesco.

Afonja, S. and Pearce T. (1986). *Social Change in Nigeria*. London: Longman.

Ake, C. (1981). *A Political Economy of Africa*. London: Longman.

Alana, E. O. (2000). "Aspects of Sorcery and Witchcraft in West Africa" in *West African Religious Traditions*. Ilega, D. I. (Ed.) Ado Ekiti: Hamaz Global Ventures.

Awolalu, J. D. and Dopamu, P. A. (1979). *West African Traditional Religion*. Ibadan: Onibonoje Publishers.

Baum, R. (1999). *Shrines of Slave Trade*. New York: Oxford University Press.

Bascom, W. R. and Herskovits, O. (1959). *Continuity and Change in African Culture*. Chicago: University of Chicago Press.

Basden, G. T. (1938). *Niger Igbo*. London: Frank Cass and Co. Ltd.

Bassey, E. O. (n.d.). *Who is this Man Olumba Olumba Obu*. Calabar: Brotherhood Press.

Bedd, N. W. and Vogel, E. E. (1963). *A Modern Introduction of the Family*. New York: Free Press.

Bevan, E. (1962). *Symbolism and Belief*. London: Fontana Library.

Beattie, J. (1963). "Sorcery in Buyoro" in J. Middleton and E. H. Winter (Eds) *Witchcraft and Sorcery in East Africa*. London: Routledge and Kegan Paul.

Commaroff, J. and Commaroff. J. L. (1993). *Modernity and its Malcontents*. Chicago: The University of Press.

de Waal Malefijit, A. (1968). *Religion and Culture: An Introduction to Anthropology*. London: Macmillan.

Dhavamony, M. (1973). *The Phenomenology of Religion Documental Missionalia-7*. Rome: Gregorian University Press.

Dickson, K. and llingworth, P. (Ed) (1969). *Biblical Revelation and African Beliefs* London: Lutterworth Press.

Donoram, W. O. (1992). *Biblical Christianity in African Perspective.* London: Paternoster Press.

Dopamu, A. and Awolalu, J. O. (1979). *West African Traditional Religion.* Ibadan: Onibonoje Press.

Ekong E. (1979). *The Sociology of the Ibibio.* Calabar: Scholar's Press.

Eliade, M. (1961). *Images and Symbols.* London: Harvill Press.

Evans-Pritchard, E. E. (1966). *Theories of Primitive Religions.* Oxford: Claredon Press.

Evans-Pritchard, E. E. (1976). *Witchcraft, Oracle and Medicine among the Azande.* Oxford: Claredon Press.

Fawcett, T. (1970). *The Symbolic Language of Religion.* London: S. C. M. Press.

Field, M. J. (1937). *Religion and Medicine of the Ga People.* London: Oxford University Press.

Field, M. J. (1960). *Search for Security: An Ethno Psychiatric Study of Rural Ghana.* London: Faber and Faber.

Frazer, J. G. (1973). *The Golden Bough: A Study in Medicine and Religion.* (3rd Ed.), Vol. II, Hong Kong: Macmillam Press.

Haralambos, M. (1980). *Sociology: Themes and Perspectives* Slough: University Tutorial Press.

Harwood, A. (1970) *Witchcraft, Sorcery and Social Categories Among the Safwa.* Oxford: Oxford University Press.

Horton, R. (1980). *Pattern of Though in Africa and the West.* London: Cambridge University Press.

Idowu, E. B. (1975). *African Traditional Religion: A Definition.* London: S.C.M. Press.

Ilega, D. I. (2001). "The Urhobo People and Witchcraft Belief" in *Journal of Religion and Culture*, vol 3 No 2.

Illogu, E. (1974). *Christianity and Ibo Culture.* Leiden: E. J. Brill.

Ikenga, M. E. (1981). *God and Man in Africa Religion*. London: Geoffrey Chapman.

Ikenga, M. E. (1987). *Comparative Studies of African Traditional Religions*. Onitsha: Imico Publishers.

Ikenga, M. E. (1986). *The Gods in Retreats: Continuity and Change in Africa Religion*. Enugu: Fourth Dimension Publishers.

Ikenga, M. E. (1985). *Africa Religion in Western Conceptual Schemes* Ibadan: Pastoral Institute, Bodija.

Ilega, D. I. (Ed). (2001). *Studies in Word Religions*. Ekiti: Hamaz Global Publishers.

Jacob, D. A. (2007). "Witchcraft Belief and Practice Among Epie /Atiss People" Unpublished M.A. Thesis, department of religious and Cultural Studies, School of Graduate Studies, University of Port Harcourt, Port Harcourt.

Kalu, O. U. (Ed). (1978). *Readings in Africa Humanities: African Cultural Development*. Enugu: Fourth Dimension.

Kinsley, M. (1964). *West Africa Studies*. London: Frank Cass and Co.

Langer, S. (1960). *Philosophy in a New Key*. Mass: Cambridge University Press.

Lehmann, A. C. and J. E. Meyer. (2000). *Magic, Witchcraft and Religion: An Anthropological Study of the Supernatural*. New York: McGraw Hill Publishers.

Malinowski, B. (1970). *Crime and Custom in Savage Society*. London: Routledge and Kegan Paul.

Mbiti, J. S. (1969). *African Religion and Philosophy* London: Heinemann.

Mbiti, J. S. (1975). *Introduction to African Religion*. London: Heinemann.

Middleton, J. and Winter, E. H. (Eds) (1963). *Witchcraft and Sorcery in East Africa*, London: Routledge and Kengan Paul.

Mume, J. O. (n.d). *Traditional Medicine in Nigeria*. Agbarho: JOM Curative Centre.

Nadel, S. F. (1954). *Nupe Religion*. London. Routledge and Kengan Paul.

Ndiokwere, N. I. (1981). *Prophecy and Revolution: The Role of Prophets in the Independent Africa Churches and in Biblical Tradition.* London: Camelot Press.

Neal, I. E. (1958). *Juju in My Life.* London: Frank Cass.

Noss, J. B. (1963). *Man's Religions.* London: Collier, Macmillan.

Nzimiro, I. (1972). *Studies in Ibo Political Systems.* London: Frank Cass.

Offiong, D. (1991). *Magic and Social Order Among the Ibibio of Nigeria:* Enugu: Dimension Publisher.

Okorocha, C. (1987). *The Meaning of Religious Conversion is Africa: The Case of Igbo of Nigeria.* Vermont: Avebury Gower.

Okot, P'Bitek. (1971). *African Religions in Western Scholarship.* Nairobi: East African Literature Bureau.

Okaba, B.O. (1997). *Why Nigerians Bury Their Money.* Choba: EMHAI Printing & Co.

Olusakin, V. A. (2013). "Sorcery and Witchcraft: An Aspect of African Science" in *An Introduction to African Culture and Technology Development;* Owete, K.I. (Ed). Port Harcourt. University of Port Harcourt Press.

Ottenberg, S. (1959). *Ibo Receptivity to Change: Continuity and Change in Africa Cultures.* Chicago: University of Chicago Press.

Parrinder, G. (1969). *Africa Religions.* London: Sheldon Press.

Parrinder, G. (1965). *African Traditional Religions.* London: Sheldon Press.

Radecliffe-Brown, A. R. (1952). *Structure and Function in Primitive Society* London: Cohen and West.

Ranger, T. O. and Kimambo, I. N. (Ed.) (1972). *The Historical Study of Africa Religion.* California: California University Press.

Rives W. H. R. (1925). *Medicine, Medicine and Religions* London: Kegan Paul Trench Trubner and Co.

Scanzoni L and Scanzoni J. (1976). *Men Women and Change A Sociology of Marriage and Family.* New York: Mc Graw Hill.

Shorter, A. (1975). *African Christian Theology*. London: Geoffrey Chapman.

Smith, R. (1974). *Ancestor Worship in Contemporary Japan*. California: Stanford University Press.

Sofowora, A. (1984). *Medicinal Plants and Traditional Medicine in Africa*. Ibadan: Spectrum Books.

Temple, P. (1959). *Bantu Philosophy*. Paris: Presence Africanies.

Trimigham, J. S. (1955). *The Christian Church and Islam in West Africa*. London: SMC Press.

Turner, V. M. (1970). *The Forest of Symbols: Aspect of Ndembu Ritual*. London: Cornell University Press.

Turner, V. M. (1965). *The Drums of Affiction: A Study of Religious Processes among the Ndembu of Zambia:* Oxford: Clarendon Press.

Ubrurhe, J. O. (2003). *Urhobo Traditional Medicine*. Ibadan: Spectrum Books.

Vetter, G. B. (1959). *Medicine and Religion: Their Psychological Nature, Origin and function*. London: Vision Press Limited.

Weber, M. (1930). *The Protestant Ethic and The Spirit of Capitalism*. London: Allen and Urwin.

Weber, H. (1948). *Medicine: A Sociological Study*. Stanford: California University Press.

Westerman, D. (1976). *African and Christianity*. London: Oxford University Press.

Whitehead, A. N. (1960). *Symbolism: Its Meaning and Effect*. Cambridge: Cambridge University Press.

Wilson, M. (1971). *Religion and Transformation of Society*. Cambridge: Cambridge University Press.

Wilson, M. (1957). *Rituals of Kinship among the Nyakusa*. London: Oxford University Press.

Journals

Ejizu C. I. (1989). "Religion and Social Change. The Case of the Igbo of Nigeria". *Neue Zeitschrift Fun Missionwissenschaft (NZM)*. Vol. 4, No. 2, pp. 112–120.

Firth, R. (1950). "Religious Belief and Personal Adjustment", *Journal of Royal Anthropological Institute*, pp. 78–81.

Fortes, M. (n.d.) "Pictals in Ancestor Worship". *Journal of Royal Anthropological Institute.* Vol. 92/2, pp. 38–44.

Horton, R. (1972). "Spiritual Beings and Elementary Particles", 2nd *Order* vol. 1, no.1, pp. 17–25.

Horton, R. (1971). "African Conversion". *Africa.* Vol. 42, No.2, pp 26–34.

Horton, R. (1962). "The Kalabari Word View: An Outline and Interpretation", *Africa.* Vol. 32, pp. 14–20.

Idowu, E. B (1971). "Witchcraft", in The Traditional Background to Medical Practice in Nigeria, Institute of African Studies Occasional Publications. No. 25, pp. 34–39.

Ikenga, M. E. (n.d.). "Implication of a Phenomenological Approach to the Study of African Religious", *Bulletin of Religion*, University of Salisbury, pp. 12–20.

Ikenga, M. E. (n.d.). "Search for Methodology of African Religion". *Journal of West African Religion,* University of Nigeria, pp. 20–26.

Otubanjo, F. (1987). "Understanding Rituals". *Orita* Ibadan: *Journal of Religious Studies* XX/I June pp. 18–22.

Turner, H. (1981). "The Way Forward in the Study of African Primal Religions". *Journal of Religion in Africa.* Vol. XII.

Encyclopaedias

Hastings, J. (Ed.) (1912). *Encyclopaedias for Religion and Ethics.* Vol. 4. Edinburgh: T and T. Clark, Morrison and Gibb.

Encyclopaedias Americana, International Ed. (1929). Vol. 19. Danbury Connecticut Americana.

Robison, M. *et.al* (Eds) (1996). *Chamber* 21st *Century Dictionary.*

Onions, C. T. (Ed) (1982). *Shorter Oxford English Dictionary.* Vol. 11, London: Oxford University Press.

Unpublished Materials

Dopamu, D. A. (1977). "Medicine in Yoruba Traditional Religion". University of Ibadan, Ph.D Thesis.

Horton, R. (1984). "Ojoye Adum" Lecture Notes.

Iwegbue, S. O. (1981). "The Origin and Organization of Anglican Mission in Ndokwa Local Government Area of Bendel State". University of Ibadan. Unpublished B.A. Long Essay.

Kayode, J. O. (1975). "Symbology with Particular Reference to the Religion of the Yoruba". University of Ibadan, Ph.D Thesis.

Okeke, E. O. (1982). "Religious Change in Ikenanzi, C.1700–1930: A Study of Growth in the Traditional Religion and Impact of Christianity". Unpublished M.A. Thesis, Department of History, Faculty of Humanities, University of Port Harcourt.

Owete, K. I. (1990). Medicine Beliefs and Practices in Emu, A Town in Ndokwa West L.G.A. of Delta State. Unpublished M.A., Thesis, Department of Religious Studies, Faculty of Arts, University of Jos.

Appendices

Appendix I

Primary Source: Oral Testimony and People Intervewed

No	Name	Age	Status	Date	Place of Interview
1	Abanum Oliver	40	Medicine man	5/9/1990	Emu
2	Abigide Ikweke	45	Medicine man	6/9/1990	Emu
3	A. Chukwukenum	68	Medicine man	1/9/1990	Emu
4	Enyabine	65	Rtd. Vice principal	8/9/1987	Emu
5	Ifeaka Odinama	60	Medicine man	5/9/1990	Emu
6	Iloma Uzor	96	Founding member of the Roman Catholic Church, Emu	3/4/1988	Emu
7	Idonor, Isakpa	102	Traditionalworshipper and *Ada*	23/8/1997	Emu
8	Isakpa, Omenogor	115	Medicine man	7/9/1987	Emu
9	Maledo	67	Rtd. Headmaster	5/9/1987	Emu
10	Nwabefa Peter	51	Medicine man	29/8/1990	Emu
11	Odalue Chukwudi	64	Medicine man	3/9/1990	Emu
12	Okoligwu Peter	61	Rt. Teacher	12/8/1990	Emu
13	Okponku Adams	52	Businessman	2/8/1990	Emu
14	Onyenajua Odu,	95	Member, *Okwa* Age group	10/9/1987	Emu
15	Onyenajua Iwemdi	40	Lay medicine man	7/9/1990	Emu
16	Iwegbue, Onyebak	47	Lectuer	28/8/9/10/1987	Abraka/ Emu
17	Oshilim Chijioke	48	Medicine man	28/7/1990	Emu
18	Oshinwa Uche	55	Medicine man	4/9/1990	Emu
19	Ossai Ijeoma	60	Medicine man	2/9/1990	Emu
20	Uwaenyashi, C.	65	Medicine man	30/9/1990	Emu
21	Peter Onuosa	47	Medicine man & and priest of *Ikenga*	2/9/2003	Emu
22	Iyama Oguise	73	Medicine man	1/9/2003	Emu
23	Patrick Enuademu	53	Medicine man, *Onotu* of Emu, Assistant priest of *Nze*	31/8/2003	Emu
24	Patrick Dibe Odili	79	*Oyiwa* of Emu	30/8/2003	Emu

No	Name	Age	Status	Date	Place of Interview
25	Johenny Enwemike	46	Traditionalist, *Onotu* of Emu, priest of *Ikenga*	29/8/2003	Emu
26	George Dakwa	68	Traditionalist	30/9/2003	Emu
27	Ikusama Abanum	92	*Okpala-ukwu* (ikosa)	2/9/2003	Emu
28	Okeleka Akabue	94	*Okpala-ukwu* (Ebilije)	2/9/2003	Emu
29	Okobi Owete	96	*Okwa* of Emu	28/8/2003	Emu
30	Ojei Ikubese	70	Head, vigilante group	27/8/2003	Emu
31	Enuma Entabegwu	83	*Ugo* of Emu (spokesman of Emu community)	28/8/2003	Emu
32	Achuenu, E.	28	Lecturer	28/9/1990	Jos

Appendix 2

Informants on Religious Beliefs and Ritual Practices

No	Name	Deity/Medicine/Festival	Interview-date
1	Enuma enyabegwu	*Olor, olokoto, odede, Ossai and Igba*	28/8/2003
2	Enwemike Johnny	*Nze, ikenga and Elishi*	29/8/2003
3	Enuademu Patrick	*Nez, odede, umuada, olokoto and Ani*	31/8/2003
4	Ikusama Abanum	*Elekali*	29/8/2003
5	Iyama Oguise	*Emo na liali ne esu mmalu, ikenga*	1/9/2003
6	George Dakwa	*Efo-olinwa, ukwuata*	30/8/2003
7	Okeleka Akabue	*Ogwu ashima*	2/9/2003
8	Onuosa Peter	*Aju ogwu*	2/9/2003
9	Idonor Isakpa	*Umuada*	23/8/1987
10	Odalue Chikwudi	*Ogwu Isolor Ibe Mmalu*	3/9/1990

Appendix 3

Types of Medicine

No	Ukwuani Name	Description
1	*Afia okeawuli*	Medicine for trade. It ensures success in spite of competition
2	*Aju ogwu*	Medicine to shield a person from spiritually sent poison
3	*Akonuche*	Medicine to enhance memory
4	*Akpanyaga*	Medicine to create disharmony
5	*Ashima*	Medicine that give premonition
6	*Efo-olinwa*	Medicine to cure stomach illness
7	*Egbe ufie*	Medicine that makes one invulnerable to bullets
8	*Elieligba nwata oseleka*	Medicine that immunes the user to bullets and sharp objects
9	*Emo na lialli ne esu mmalu*	Medicine to cures internal discomfort
10	*Enya enu*	Medicine to cure malady or psychosis
11	*Eti ada*	Medicine to overpower an enemy
12	*Ibo mmalu onu*	Medicine to make a victim crazy
13	*Ife mmili*	Medicine to stop rainfall
14	*Igba nkpa*	Medicine to shoot poisionous objects into a victom's body
15	*Igbele*	Medicine to cure veneral diseases and miscarriage in women
16	*Ikpofu onwu mmalu*	Medicine to postponed the death of a dying person
17	*Isorlu mmalu*	Medicine to gain the love of a person, even against their will
18	*Iwa ugboko*	Medicine to command obeisance
20	*Ogwu Mma*	Medicine that immunes the user to cutless and knife cuts
21	*Mma mbubu*	Medicine to nullify *Ogwu nma*
22	*Mmo ni mmalu afu enya*	Medicine to suspend temporarily death
23	*Nkpashi*	Medicine to warn of the presence of poison in food or drink
24	*Nkpokwa*	Medicine to prevent attack from evil medicine
25	*Njo puazu*	Medicine to teleport user from danger
26	*Udo*	Medicine to call a person back to Emus

Index

www.ingramcontent.com/pod-product-compliance
Ingram Content Group UK Ltd.
Pitfield, Milton Keynes, MK11 3LW, UK
UKHW021014120926
8556IPUK00040B/1140

9 783631 659786